Getting the Most from Nursing School: A Guide to Becoming a Nurse

Robert Atkins, PhD, RN
Assistant Professor
Rutgers, The State University of New Jersey
Newark Campus
College of Nursing

JONES AND BARTLETT PUBLISHERS
Sudbury, Massachusetts
BOSTON   TORONTO   LONDON   SINGAPORE

World Headquarters

Jones and Bartlett Publishers	Jones and Bartlett Publishers	Jones and Bartlett Publishers
40 Tall Pine Drive	Canada	International
Sudbury, MA 01776	6339 Ormindale Way	Barb House, Barb Mews
978-443-5000	Mississauga, Ontario L5V 1J2	London W6 7PA
info@jbpub.com	Canada	United Kingdom
www.jbpub.com		

Jones and Bartlett's books and products are available through most bookstores and online booksellers. To contact Jones and Bartlett Publishers directly, call 800-832-0034, fax 978-443-8000, or visit our website www.jbpub.com.

Substantial discounts on bulk quantities of Jones and Bartlett's publications are available to corporations, professional associations, and other qualified organizations. For details and specific discount information, contact the special sales department at Jones and Bartlett via the above contact information or send an email to specialsales@jbpub.com.

The authors, editor, and publisher have made every effort to provide accurate information. However, they are not responsible for errors, omissions, or for any outcomes related to the use of the contents of this book and take no responsibility for the use of the products and procedures described. Treatments and side effects described in this book may not be applicable to all people; likewise, some people may require a dose or experience a side effect that is not described herein. Drugs and medical devices are discussed that may have limited availability controlled by the Food and Drug Administration (FDA) for use only in a research study or clinical trial. Research, clinical practice, and government regulations often change the accepted standard in this field. When consideration is being given to use of any drug in the clinical setting, the health care provider or reader is responsible for determining FDA status of the drug, reading the package insert, and reviewing prescribing information for the most up-to-date recommendations on dose, precautions, and contraindications, and determining the appropriate usage for the product. This is especially important in the case of drugs that are new or seldom used.

Production Credits

Publisher: Kevin Sullivan
Acquisitions Editor: Amy Sibley
Acquisitions Editor: Emily Ekle
Editorial Assistant: Patricia Donnelly
Editorial Assistant: Rachel Shuster
Production Assistant: Sarah Bayle
Associate Marketing Manager: Ilana Goddess
Manufacturing and Inventory Control Supervisor:
 Amy Bacus

Composition and Interior Design: Auburn Associates, Inc.
Cover Design: Kristin E. Ohlin
Cover Image: © Dewayne Flowers/Shutterstock, Inc.
Printing and Binding: Malloy, Inc.
Cover Printing: Malloy, Inc.

Library of Congress Cataloging-in-Publication Data
Atkins, Robert, M.S.
 Getting the most from nursing school : a guide to becoming a nurse / Robert Atkins. — 1st ed.
  p. ; cm.
 Includes bibliographical references and index.
 ISBN-13: 978-0-7637-5581-2 (alk. paper)
 ISBN-10: 0-7637-5581-8 (alk. paper)
 1. Nursing. 2. Nursing—Vocational guidance. I. Title.
 [DNLM: 1. Education, Nursing. 2. Career Choice. 3. Students, Nursing. WY 18 A874g 2009]
 RT71.A85 2009
 610.7306'9—dc22
                              2008011324

6048

Printed in the United States of America
12 11 10 09 08   10 9 8 7 6 5 4 3 2 1

DEDICATION

For my sons R.J. and Pierce

TABLE OF CONTENTS

PREFACE

Why Did I Write This Book?

One reason I decided to write this book was that I would have been better off if I had one like it when I was contemplating going to nursing school and when I was in the process of applying to nursing school. I didn't really know what I was getting myself into, and I remember I had a number of questions about nursing school and the profession of nursing: Would I be better off going to medical school? What is the difference between an associate degree program in nursing and a baccalaureate degree program in nursing? Should I apply to a BSN–MSN program? How does one become a nurse practitioner? I was fortunate in that I knew several experienced nurses (like my mother) who could share their thoughts on these questions; however, while I appreciated their thoughts, I would have loved to have had the perspective of other insiders such as professors or leaders in the profession (similar to the way that I like to ask food servers at a restaurant for their recommendations when ordering). Unfortunately, at the time, I did not know many nursing insiders. The recommendations in this guide come from the knowledge and experience of insiders I have met since I began my career in nursing.

I also wrote this book because I regret that I did not make the most of my learning opportunities in nursing school. I had the good fortune to be accepted to the Accelerated Bachelor of Science in Nursing program at the

University of Pennsylvania's School of Nursing, where I was taught by nationally renowned researchers and expert clinicians; however, I approached my studies with the intention of "surviving" rather than making the most of my time at one of the best nursing programs in the United States (and probably the world). I have come to realize that because I approached nursing school with the same mindset I would if I were faced with an oncoming tornado or a shark attack ("I just want to live to see tomorrow"), I developed a strong dislike of nursing school. In fact, I have often said, "I love being a nurse, but I hated nursing school." If I had approached nursing school with the mindset that I advocate in this book, I would have learned more in nursing school and, while I am happy with what I have been able to do as a nurse, maybe I would have been able to do more had I gotten more out of nursing school.

Another motivation for writing this book is that I want to help nursing school students who are struggling. Every semester that I have taught nursing students, a few have come to me because nursing school is not going well. The reasons usually include failing grades on exams or assignments, difficulties with time management, or adversarial relationships with faculty. In most cases, these difficulties threaten the students' progress in nursing school. The contents of this book are aimed at helping these students "turn it around" and become more successful in nursing school. Included in this book is the advice that nursing professors like myself give students who are struggling. I do not propose that simply reading this book guarantees that every student will succeed in nursing; however, I do feel that what is discussed in this book will enhance and expand what most students learn in nursing school.

An additional reason for writing this book is that, although there are other books written by nurses and nonnurses that provide recommendations on how to get through nursing school, the recommendations in those books are based on anecdotes and opinions from the authors and nurses and nursing students interviewed by the authors. This book is different from those books in two distinct ways. First, while anecdotes and opinions can be useful, as a nurse and a researcher, I know the value of using evidence based on peer-reviewed research to guide decisions. Consequently, in this book I have endeavored to make sure that, whenever possible, I provide recommendations that are empirically grounded (based on scientific research and/or theoretical evidence) and supported by those who have experience teaching nursing students. As reflected in the number of citations throughout the text, in writing this book I consulted a wide variety of scholarly sources from disciplines such as nursing, education, and psychology.

Another way that this book is distinct from other nursing texts is that I interviewed nursing insiders while writing this book. While the recommendations of former and current nursing school students included in other books on nursing school are valuable, most of these individuals do not have enough experience and knowledge of nursing school and nursing to provide recommendations that are based on the "big picture." The recommendations provided in this book come from nursing faculty and nurses who have decades of experience as nurses and nursing educators. They have seen the substantial changes that nursing and nursing education have undergone in that time and, thus are well positioned to provide recommendations that will help students get the most out of their nursing education.

The final reason that I will share for writing this book is that I love being a nurse, and I care about the profession of nursing. Moreover, I strongly believe that persuading individuals who have the potential to become great nurses to enter nursing will not only improve the profession of nursing but will also improve the nation's healthcare system. Nurses outnumber all other healthcare professionals in the healthcare system, and by providing excellent care, shaping policy, educating patients and providers, and conducting meaningful research, nurses have the most potential of any healthcare provider to improve the health and well-being of this nation's citizens. To achieve these goals, nursing needs to attract more of the best and the brightest into the profession. I hope that this book will persuade those talented individuals to consider nursing and provide them with the tools to get the most out of nursing school and to become excellent care providers, policy makers, educators, and researchers.

More on Why Nursing and Society Need the Best and Brightest

There are a few books available to students that take a "survival guide approach" to nursing school; however, that approach does nothing for the profession of nursing. More importantly, the survival guide approach to nursing school is not in the best interest of healthcare consumers. Indeed, nurses take care of people's loved ones—their infants, parents, wives, brothers, neighbors, and college roommates—and all of these people deserve more than someone who just survived nursing school. The world needs nurses who are clinically skilled, compassionate, and committed to learning as much as possible because they know that their knowledge, skills, and compassion are sometimes the difference between life and death.

How do excellent nurses make the difference between what ought to happen in the healthcare system and what happens too often in the healthcare system? Below are several real world examples:

Mrs. Smith, a pregnant woman, arrives with her husband and is admitted to the hospital in labor with what will be their first child. All goes well with the labor and delivery process, and Mrs. Smith gives birth vaginally to a healthy baby boy. After the birth, the typical procedures are performed: mucus is removed from the newborn's nose, the umbilical cord is cut, and the baby is given a brief examination before being returned to his parents.

What ought to happen: Within an hour of the birth, Mrs. Smith, who had already made the decision to breastfeed, is given an opportunity to breastfeed, and she receives education from her nurse on the benefits (e.g., health benefits to the baby and the mother, financial benefits) of breastfeeding. The nurse provides more education, support, and encouragement when Mrs. Smith's initial attempts to breastfeed are not successful and arranges for her to have an appointment with the lactation nurse (nurse with special training in breastfeeding) before discharge. The nurse also makes sure that discharge instructions include information on breastfeeding and community resources such as the La Leche League. After discharge, Mrs. Smith continues to breastfeed for the next 6 months: a breastfeeding success story.

What happens too often: Assuming that the mother does not want to breastfeed— and too busy or distracted with other tasks to discuss breastfeeding with her patient—the nurse asks Mrs. Smith, "What type of formula would you prefer?" Mrs. Smith gives up on her plan to breastfeed.

Mr. Jordan is a 65-year-old patient on the orthopedic rehabilitation floor for a hip replacement. His recent medical history is remarkable for a previous hospitalization in which he stopped breathing or had respiratory arrest. After three days on the orthopedic rehabilitation floor, he begins to complain of respiratory distress. Mr. Jordan appears anxious as he explains to his primary nurse that the last time he felt like this was when he stopped breathing. His primary nurse does a physical assessment and collects vital signs: his blood pressure is 102/62 (lower than usual for him), his respiratory rate is 30 (a little faster than usual), and his pulse rate is 140 (much faster than usual). Following hospital protocol, she calls the medical intern and a respiratory therapist. The intern performs a physical exam and reassures the patient that "You will be alright," at which point the respiratory therapist packs up and leaves the patient's room.

What ought to happen: The primary nurse should share her concerns with the intern and explain that Mr. Jordan should be transferred off of the orthopedic rehabilitation floor and to an intensive care unit. In turn, the intern should write an order to have Mr. Jordan transferred. If that does not happen, the nurse should call the attending physician and report that the intern examined the patient and determined that the patient was stable, but you feel that the patient is at risk to go into respiratory arrest. In turn, the attending physician should give the nurse a verbal order to transfer the patient to the critical care unit for observation, where the likelihood of averting or managing a life-threatening event are much better than on a medical–surgical floor.

What happens too often. The primary nurse decides not to express her concerns and goes along with the intern's decision. She reassures the patient that he will feel better in a few hours. An hour later she enters the room to find Mr. Jones gasping for air and with a blue pallor. She initiates a code and begins CPR. The code team arrives in less than one minute, but they are unable to resuscitate Mr. Jones.

Ms. Lopez presented to the emergency department with her two-year-old son Jesus and her five-year-old son Hector. Hector fell of his bicycle earlier in the day and injured his arm, which had become increasingly swollen and bruised. His nurse in the emergency department gathers information from the mother regarding Hector, such as his past medical history, history of present illnesses, and known allergies. In discussing Hector's health history, Ms. Lopez mentions that Jesus, her two-year-old, "doesn't say much." Ms. Lopez goes on to explain that Jesus "uses less language than his cousins who are the same age." In fact, he often just points to things that he wants. Ms. Lopez reports that her pediatrician told her not to worry, that Jesus was "just a late bloomer"; however, she admits that she is starting to worry and is "unsure what I should do."

What ought to happen. The emergency department nurse takes a few minutes to gather history on Jesus (e.g., birth, developmental, illness) and provide education to Ms. Lopez on speech and language development in toddlers (e.g., most children Jesus's age are combining words). While Hector is waiting for his X-rays to be read, the nurse gives Ms. Lopez information on the early intervention program (EIP) and assists her in calling EIP for an evaluation of Jesus.

Jesus receives a speech and language evaluation through EIP that shows mild receptive and expressive language delay after the diagnosis and treatment of a middle ear effusion and a hearing test. Jesus begins weekly speech and language therapy, and at age three, he starts receiving speech and language services through his public school system, where he continues to make progress in his speech and language development. At the start of kindergarten Jesus is indistinguishable from his peers in terms of language, behavior, and cognitive ability.

What happens too often. The emergency department nurse reassures Ms. Lopez that Jesus is probably a "late bloomer." The nurse adds that he "has a cousin who did not start speaking until he was five." Jesus's speech and language continue to develop more slowly than his peers', and it is not until he reaches kindergarten that he is formally evaluated for hearing loss. Because of how late he receives speech and language services, Jesus lags behind his peers academically and displays more behavioral problems (e.g., aggressive behavior, inattentiveness) than his peers.

As illustrated by these scenarios, excellent nurses can make a big difference in the health outcomes of patients simply by doing for patients what one would want done for a member of his or her own family. The nurse's actions described in each of the *what ought to happen* scenarios are consonant with what we would want done for our loved ones and what the research suggests exemplifies excellence in nursing. For example, in a qualitative study conducted to understand excellence in nursing, Coulon and colleagues (1996) found that in addition to being competent and compassionate, nurses judged by other nurses as being excellent kept the patient (and family) always as the primary focus of their concern.

In contrast, the nurse's actions described in each of the *what happens too often* scenarios suggest that other factors (e.g., time pressures, confidence) interfered with doing what was best for the patient. It is important to point out that the nurse's actions described in the *what happens too often* scenarios would probably not be considered malpractice: the nurse in these scenarios did nothing that would merit disciplinary action or spark litigation. However, as will be discussed in this book, society needs nurses who do more than stay out of legal trouble. By committing yourself to getting the most out of nursing school, you take a first step toward becoming an excellent nurse.

What Can Nursing Do for You?

One reason I love being a nurse is that, while I regret that I did not take full advantage of my time in nursing school, my nursing education (formal and informal) has given me a great way to make a living, gain technical skills, and have a knowledge of health and the healthcare system I doubt I would have obtained had I pursued another profession. Moreover, nursing pushed me in a direction that helped me to become a more compassionate and more thoughtful person than I would have become otherwise. I have no scientific evidence for my claim that nursing had something to do with this development, and as they say with all of the advertisements for diet pills, "Your results may vary." However, in the section that follows I briefly discuss the personal benefits of pursuing a career in nursing.

Develop a Nursing-Inspired Worldview

One benefit of pursuing a career in nursing is that one develops a nursing-inspired worldview. What do I mean by nursing-inspired worldview? At some point in their nursing education, all nursing students begin to think about what it means to be a nurse and to provide care for others. The educational process of becoming a nurse (e.g., classroom discussions, clinical experiences, readings) influences how one thinks about nursing and providing care for others, but each individual will come to his or her own personal way of thinking about nursing. This way of thinking will not only guide one's nursing practice and how one provides care, but this thinking will also affect how one views the world.

For example, the process of thinking about what it means to be a nurse and to provide care for others made me come to the simple realization that no one on this planet wants to suffer—by suffering I mean illnesses, conditions, and circumstances that result in physical, emotional, and spiritual pain. I realized that no one wants to be impoverished, obese, drug-addicted, homeless, selfish, or depressed: everyone is doing the best they can with the resources (social, physical, economic, intellectual) they have, and as a nurse and fellow human being, I have to accept them for who they are or assist them in increasing their resources.

I am not arguing that my nursing-inspired worldview has inoculated me against becoming frustrated with those who engage in behaviors that diminish their health and well-being, because it has not. However, my nursing-inspired worldview helped me to be more caring and thoughtful when I worked with a middle-aged man who was in kidney failure but missed his last three appointments with his nephrologists, or when I counseled the 14-year-old female who said that she did not want to get pregnant but continued to have unprotected sex. I realized that I was not helping these individuals by focusing on *what* they were doing or not doing to get healthy. I needed to focus on *why* they were not doing what was in their best interest.

The Skills That One Develops in Nursing School

In addition to thinking like a nurse and developing a nursing-inspired worldview, through the process of becoming a nurse you will develop certain skills that give you an advantage over most people who are not nurses. In the section below I discuss some of the fundamental skills that you develop in nursing school.

The Ability to Manage Time

A skill all successful nurses develop is the ability to manage time. The ability to manage time is probably valuable in many professions but in nursing it is indispensable or *sine qua non* (Latin for "without which it could not be"). For example, in a study of 26 nurses in nine different hospitals, one researcher found in a typical eight-hour shift, nurses cared for an average of six patients and they completed 160 tasks with an average task time of 168 seconds (Wiggins, 2006). Most of these tasks—which include patient-centered activities such as providing education, dispensing medication, and assessing patients—are complex and require a combination of critical thinking, psychomotor, and interpersonal skills.

The Ability to Prioritize

One reason that most successful nurses are such good time managers is they have learned to prioritize. In nursing and other healthcare domains, the concept of prioritizing is referred to as *triage*, which means "to sort" in French. The concept of triage in the medical domain emerged on the battlefield and referred specifically to prioritizing patients and providing immediate care to the most seriously injured. Learning to triage is also a big part of thinking like a nurse. Like healthcare providers engaged in battlefield or disaster triage, nurses have to make assessments of patients and resources to determine what has to be done first and what can wait until later. For most individuals, the process of learning to think in this manner begins in nursing school. From the first clinical rotation, students begin to learn how to triage and figure out how to make the most of scarce resources. While nursing students are typically not making life-and-death decisions, they have to prioritize the care they will provide. In the first clinical experience the nursing student only has responsibility for one patient, but that is difficult for most as they have to decide what they should do first—pass medications, begin discharge teaching for the patient in Room 212, or answer the call light in Room 216. With each clinical week the process of triaging their clinical resources becomes more complex as student nurses become responsible for more patients and they have to make more clinical decisions.

The Ability to Make Systematic Assessments

Another valuable skill that one gets from a nursing education, which is related to time management and triaging, is the ability to quickly assess patients systematically. Anyone can quickly assess a patient ("looks okay to me"); however, nurses learn to evaluate patients systematically, and this increases the likelihood that evaluations will be accurate. Learning to make systematic health assessments begins in nursing school, where students learn pathophysiological principles, how to perform comprehensive health histories and head-to-toe physical examinations, and to distinguish normal and abnormal variations.

During nursing school, nursing students also begin to develop the skills to detect signs that something is wrong and immediate action is warranted—an essential component of systematic evaluation that develops with knowledge and experience. These signs are often referred to as "red flags." As part of our education, all nurses have clinical experiences in acute care settings where, despite the fact that a great number of tasks have to be completed in a short amount of time, we learn the importance of assessing patients at every opportunity because patients can deteriorate quickly. Because it would not be practical or possible to do a comprehensive physical health exam on a patient in the acute care setting on an hourly basis, nurses learn to assess patients during routine interactions with the patient throughout the shift, such as administering medications or providing education, and these assessments include evaluating the patient for red flags (e.g., slurring of speech, shortness of breath).

I can still clearly recall a red flag I picked up while working in an acute care setting shortly after graduating from nursing school. As I walked past a female patient in her early 60s sitting in a wheelchair near the nurses' station, a voice in my head said, "Something is not right with her color; she looks gray." A quick assessment of the patient (vital signs, pulse oximetry) indicated that she was "crashing" and in danger of cardiopulmonary arrest. I called what is referred to in some hospitals as a "code," which alerts a specially trained team of providers (nurses, physicians, respiratory therapists) to rush to a specific location—in this case my floor—and begin resuscitative efforts. The patient was resuscitated and transferred to the intensive care unit, where she recovered.

How Nursing Has Helped Me Outside of My Work as a Nurse

Time management, triaging, and the ability to make systematic and accurate assessments are indispensable to success in the profession of nursing, but these skills are also useful outside of nursing. In my life outside of nursing as a researcher, a worker in the community, and a parent, my experiences in nursing have come in handy. For example, as a researcher I am always facing some deadline, such as a funding proposal that has to be submitted or a journal article that has to be revised. In fact, there is always something that I could (should?) be writing, reading, or revising. This constant stream of deadlines could make life nerve-wracking; however, my nursing education and experiences have helped me to keep the work in perspective. As a nurse I have learned to take what seems like a large, unmanageable task (e.g., preparing a 25-page funding proposal to the National Institutes of Health) and breaking it into smaller more manageable tasks (e.g., writing up the analytical plan for the 25-page funding proposal). In this way I am able to move past the paralysis that sometimes sets in when one is faced with the challenge of accomplishing a range of tasks in a fixed amount of time.

Nursing has also taught me to prioritize by asking the question, "What has to be done right now and what can wait?" Taking the time to answer this question is almost always worth it. For example, my wife works some evenings and weekends (as a nurse), so I get to be head of the household when she is out of the house. I would probably enjoy this elevation in household status more if not for the fact that in my role as head of the household I am solely responsible for the care and well-being of our two young sons: R.J. and Pierce. Because these two boys are very active, I find myself faced with numerous decisions in which I have to prioritize: Clean up after dinner or take the boys to the park while it is still light out? Fix the flat tire on Pierce's bike or play with R.J. on the trampoline? Get Pierce off the toilet or get R.J. into the shower? See why R.J. is crying in the backyard or why Pierce is crying in the front yard? Thinking like a nurse keeps me sane and allows me to make the most of a scarce resource (me) as I try to meet the needs of my sons.

Overview of the Text

The first five chapters of this book are devoted to helping potential nurses think about nursing and nursing school. In the first chapter, I discuss some of the most commonly voiced reasons individuals provide for deciding against nursing or nursing school. Provided in Chapter 2 is a primer on how one becomes a registered nurse. In Chapter 3, I pull back the curtains on the nursing school institution and give readers an understanding of how it is set up and what they should know about the persons who work there (e.g., faculty, administrators). In Chapter 4, I discuss how to get into nursing school. Each year tens of thousands of qualified students are denied admission to nursing school; consequently, the importance of assembling the best possible admission application cannot be overemphasized. Finally, in Chapter 5, I provide a brief overview and description of the courses one is required to take as a nursing student.

Beginning in Chapter 6, the focus of the book turns to helping nursing school students make the most of their time in nursing school. In Chapter 6, recommendations are provided on how to establish a productive rapport with the faculty members who guide the education of nursing students. In Chapter 7, I discuss evidence-based strategies for optimizing what one gets out of the nursing school courses through activities such as attending class, taking notes systematically, and reading with a purpose. A growing number of institutions offer courses online, and in Chapter 8, I provide some recommendations on how to optimize learning on the information superhighway. As nursing students and nurses, it is important to be able to present information both orally and in written form; accordingly, readers are provided guidance on how to make oral presentations in Chapter 9 and to write papers in nursing school in Chapter 10. In Chapter 11, I provide a brief discussion of plagiarism and academic dishonesty. Chapter 12 deals with the clinical experience; readers are provided with guidance on how to optimize the clinical experiences they will undergo as nursing school students. As noted, the ability to manage time is an indispensable nursing skill, and in Chapter 13 discussion on how to develop this skill is provided. In Chapter 14, evidence-based strategies for taking tests in nursing school are provided. Finally, the appendix includes additional recommendations and anecdotes that I gathered from the interviews I conducted in the course of writing this book.

Features of the Text

- Insider information—In addition to reviewing the literature from disciplines such as nursing, education, and psychology in the writing of this book, I conducted interviews with nursing insiders such as nursing faculty members and other experienced nurses who have worked closely with nursing students. These individuals provided valuable insights and recommendations on topics such as handling the pressures of clinical rotations and poignant anecdotes of experiences in nursing and nursing school.

- Recommendations for nontraditional populations in nursing school— Although most of the insights, recommendations, and anecdotes offered in this book will benefit students from all backgrounds, the interviewees for this book also provided recommendations meant to assist individuals who do not fit the traditional profile of nursing school students (e.g., English-speaking, female, under the age of 25) to get the most out of nursing school. These nontraditional students include men, parents, and students for whom English is a second language.

- Real-world illustrations—Another feature of the text is (in addition to evidence-based information on getting the most out of nursing school) the inclusion of examples of papers, presentations, and questions that illustrate the strategy or concept being discussed. For example, in Chapter 10, which is about writing a paper in nursing school, a paper from a former student has been included with my critique indicating how the student adhered to or deviated from the recommendations discussed in the book. In Chapter 4, in which I focus on getting admitted to nursing school, I critiqued an admissions essay submitted by a student.

References

Coulon, L., Mok, M., Krause, K. L., & Anderson, M. (1996). The pursuit of excellence in nursing care: What does it mean? *Journal of Advanced Nursing, 24*, 817–826.

Kitson, A. (1997). Developing excellence in nursing practice and care. *Nursing Standard, 12*, 33–37.

Wiggins, M. S. (2006). The partnership care delivery model. *The Journal of Nursing Administration, 36*(7–8), 341–345.

ACKNOWLEDGMENTS

There are several people without whom I never would have written this book. I'd first like to thank my dad, Bill, the first and best role model I have had, and my mother, Betty, a great role model in addition to being the best nurse I know. You have provided unwavering support, sage advice, and encouragement to me since bringing me into the world and I am grateful. I am also grateful for the advice and support of my longtime mentor, close friend, and collaborator, Dan Hart, who has contributed to my development as a scholar (and cynical optimist) and more importantly to my development as a friend, father, and husband. You are one of the best people that I know and your friendship has been one of the most valuable gifts I have received as an adult. Last, but not least, I am deeply indebted to my beautiful and loving wife, Joy, who is a great mother to our boys and a close friend to me. You help to ease life's hurts and to amplify life's pleasures.

In addition to the support of my friends and family, I wish to acknowledge the invaluable contributions made by my colleagues in the College of Nursing at Rutgers University and other nursing programs, who provided the numerous Sidebars, Reflections, and Real-World Snapshots included in this book; these features will guide readers to get the most out of nursing school. All of the educators who contributed to this book were recruited to participate because of their reputations as excellent nurse educators committed to supporting and nurturing students.

Kathy Abel, MSN, RN
Adjunct Lecturer, College of Nursing
Rutgers, The State University of New Jersey

Elizabeth Ann Atkins, MA, RN
Clinical Director
Kennedy Health System

Joy Atkins, MA, RN
Adjunct Instructor, Department of Nursing
Rutgers, The State University of New Jersey

Cynthia Ayres, PhD, RN
Assistant Professor, College of Nursing
Rutgers, The State University of New Jersey

Carol Carofiglio, PhD, RN
Nursing Faculty
Helene Fuld School of Nursing in Camden County

Patricia Coyne, MSN, RN
Instructor, Maternity Nursing
Cochran School of Nursing

Laurie Karmel, MSN, RN
Clinical Instructor, College of Nursing
Rutgers, The State University of New Jersey

Sharon Kowalchuk, RN, MA
Instructor
Cochran School of Nursing

Jane Kurz, PhD, RN
Associate Professor, Department of Nursing
Temple University

Randolph Rasch, PhD, RN
Professor and Director of the Family Nurse Practitioner Specialty
Vanderbilt University School of Nursing

Jeanne Ruggiero, PhD, RN, APN-C
Assistant Professor, College of Nursing
Seton Hall University

Henry Soehnlein, MSN, RN
Clinical Instructor, College of Nursing
Rutgers, The State University of New Jersey

Nanette Sulik, MSN, RN
Clinical Instructor, Department of Nursing
Rutgers, The State University of New Jersey

This commitment to the education of nursing students is exemplified by my colleagues Jeanne Ruggiero, who spent long hours reading and carefully editing my writing, providing thoughtful feedback, and encouraging me in the process of writing this book, and Laurie Karmel, who spent hours sharing her clinical expertise and uplifting philosophy of nursing education with me. The many accolades and awards that the two of you have received for your teaching are well deserved. I also wish to acknowledge the many nurses and nursing students—my colleagues in training—who inspired me to write this book and provided support and encouragement throughout the process. Special thanks to former students Jeremy DiCandilo, Tara Hubach, Raphaelle Ibarra, Lynne Verderese, Pilang Thach, and Paul Wilk.

Finally, I wish to thank Sarah Bayle, Tricia Donnelly, and Amy Sibley from Jones and Bartlett Publishers for all of their assistance. Your encouraging words and thoughtful feedback have made the process of writing and developing this book enjoyable and rewarding.

ONE

I've Thought About Nursing, But...

As noted, I love being a nurse, and one reason is because of what nursing has allowed me to accomplish in my career. In fact, I have a hard time imagining a profession that would have been as perfect a fit for me as nursing. Further, some of my favorite people in this world are nurses. When I speak to someone who I believe would be a good fit for nursing, I share my love of nursing because I think nurses can make such a positive difference in the lives of others. In these situations I sometimes find myself just blurting out, "You should be a nurse." Some individuals are open to my suggestions, and many of these individuals respond by telling me that they have thought about pursuing a career in nursing, but for one reason or another they are pessimistic about fulfilling this wish. The obstacles vary, and in the sections that follow I provide evidence and experience-based guidance for those who have thought about nursing but are having a hard time putting it all together.

I Don't Like Blood or Any Other Bodily Fluids (or Solids) That Are Not Mine

This is a reason commonly offered by men and women who feel they are not well suited to become a nurse. Although I can perfectly understand this

1

reason—I was not and am not a blood and guts type of guy—there are a few things you should know if you feel that you might be interested in nursing were it not for being squeamish about blood.

A Blood–Injury Phobia Is Not Uncommon

First, it is well documented that humans have a natural tendency to squirm at the sight of blood. In fact, fainting due to diminished heart rate is not unusual in medical and nursing students (Marks, 1988). For some individuals this normal squeamishness can become so intense that even minor injuries or the word *blood* can induce fear, nausea, and fainting. Individuals with this type of severe reaction are said to have a blood–injury phobia. The treatment for those with a blood–injury phobia and those with normal squeamishness is graded and prolonged self-exposure, or habituation. Habituation occurs when after a period of exposure to a stimulus, one stops responding. As Marks (1988) explained, many individuals with blood–injury phobia can use habituation to treat themselves:

> Look at a vial of blood and lurid-colored pictures of surgery and disease (placed in the bathroom and kitchen, where they will be seen often), sit in an emergency room or a place where people are giving blood, watch and hear violent films, read gory descriptions of injury and surgery, and handle needles and syringes of increasing size (p. 1209).

Of course, for individuals whose reaction to blood or injury includes fainting (and suffering injury from the act of fainting), it is important to emphasize that precautions should be taken (e.g., have a spotter, don't initiate this exposure standing on a marble floor).

You'll Probably Get Over It

My second point for those who doubt their fitness for nursing because they are squeamish about blood and bodily functions is that the process of becoming a healthcare provider takes away some of the emotional connection to the body and makes you more concerned with how blood and bodily functions connect to an individual's health. It is hard to explain; however, as you progress through nursing school and you are quickly inundated with information on the anatomy and physiology of the human body, you become fascinated by the complexity of human beings and begin to see the human body as more of a wondrous machine. Why does it matter that many healthcare students such as nurses and medical students become fascinated with the functioning of the human body? This matters because fear and queasiness is replaced by wonder. For example, when you see oil leaking underneath your car, you do not get queasy; you wonder: Is that oil coming from my car? How can I stop that leak? Can I afford a new car? That is why most nurses and other healthcare professionals, when they are in the company of other nurses and healthcare professionals, can discuss topics like vomit, poop, urine, and ear wax during a meal like they are talking about the oil in their cars or the rain that falls from the sky. The meaning and role of these substances have completely changed.

How does it change? As a student you learn that bodily fluids all serve a function in the body, and each drop of fluid can provide clues about the body's function. I know it may be difficult to appreciate now, but nursing teaches you to think like a detective, and detectives are always thinking and looking for answers. For example, after you learn that each erythrocyte (a type of blood cell) contains approximately 280 million hemoglobin molecules—giving blood its red color—you forget about the color and think of the function. Consequently, as the process of becoming a clinician takes hold, you will see blood and you will seek answers to questions: Where is that blood coming from? How do I stop the bleeding? I wonder what the hemoglobin count of that blood is?

You will see a patient's urine and wonder: I wonder if there is blood in that urine. I wonder why that urine is so dark. Maybe that is the urine of someone who is dehydrated. How can we best rehydrate that patient? Even bowel movements in their many forms (e.g., soft and well formed, loose) will look different once you become a nurse (unfortunately, the smell will not change).

Exposure to Bodily Fluids Varies

A final factor to consider regarding squeamishness is that for most nursing students their direct exposure to bodily fluids (and solids and semisolids) during nursing school is limited. Most students dissect a fetal pig in anatomy and physiology, and some of the sights and smells (e.g., formaldehyde) associated with the dissection might be slightly unpleasant for those who are squeamish; however, the dissection progresses incrementally, which allows one to acclimate gradually to the experience. The other direct exposure to bodily fluids occurs during clinical rotations. Experiences vary, but most students observe a few surgical procedures, change wound dressings, and assist with a childbirth. For the squeamish, the sights and smells may be challenging but not insurmountable.

Moreover, direct exposure to bodily fluids after nursing school depends on what type of career one pursues as a nurse. Labor and delivery nurses see all sorts of bodily fluids, but they also get to see a child enter into the world, which is pretty amazing. In contrast, school nurses (one of my first jobs out of nursing school) have minimal exposure to blood and other bodily substances: a few bloody noses and skinned knees, but the noses and knees belong to kids you care about who have come to you for help, so you will focus on the child, not the injury. Finally, there are career paths in nursing that involve little or no exposure to blood or bodily fluids, such as nursing research or nursing administration.

Everyone Tells Me I Am Smart Enough to Go to Medical School

Many would-be nurses have told me that they once considered nursing school, but they were advised to go to medical school instead. I am familiar with this obstacle. In fact if I gained 1 millimeter of vertical leaping ability for each time someone told me, "You are smart. You should be a physician," I would be able to dunk a basketball like Michael Jordan in his prime. Be assured that I am a substantial distance away from dunking the ball at all. My point is that I know firsthand that many who are interested in nursing school have heard some variation of the above advice from friends, relatives, and well-meaning acquaintances.

The Television Myth of Smart Physicians

Anyway, where do people get this idea that physicians are so smart and that nurses are not so smart? I blame television. The first smart (and kind) physician I knew was someone I met through television, and his name was Marcus Welby, MD. I was young when I first started watching Dr. Welby practice medicine, so I don't remember much more about Dr. Welby other than he was smart, kind, and tan, and that few people died under his care. However, I do remember Quincy and his sidekick Fuji. Quincy (actor Jack Klugman) was a pathologist, and he was very smart. Although not as kind as Dr. Welby, he solved medical mysteries in less than an hour, and I was

always amazed at his powers of deduction. Quincy could spend a few moments looking at the corpse and glance over the toxicology reports from the lab and be able to
inform Fuji, "She didn't die of a tumor. She was murdered." I was always impressed.

I stopped watching the smart physicians on television after *Quincy,* but I know
that they are still in great supply due to the popularity of such medical dramas as *ER,
Grey's Anatomy,* and *House.* These shows share the following characteristics:
(1) physician characters are young, dedicated, and brilliant physicians (who think like
Quincy but look like George Clooney or Angelina Jolie), and they are able to cure
every illness while spending substantial amounts of time attending to the emotional
needs of their patients; and (2) nurse characters who are usually kind and well meaning; however, their tasks are mainly to support the physicians. I would imagine if these
shows were my basis for understanding what happens in the hospital and the
nurse–physician relationship—as is the case for most people under the age of 40
who have never been ill or had a parent hospitalized—I would believe that these
shows reflect reality. Of course, the reality is much different.

Television Depicts Hospitals Filled with Doctors

In reality, nurses make up the largest single component of hospital staff and are the
primary professional providers of hospital patient care. When a patient is hospitalized in a teaching hospital, the patient will encounter physicians, medical students,
interns, and residents, but the hospital staff who will provide the majority of the care
are the nurses. The nurses will be the ones to notice whether a patient is "starting to
go bad" or deteriorating rapidly, give medications and other treatments, and provide
education and discharge planning. In short, the physicians treat the illness while the
nurse focuses on the patient.

Television gives the impression that great doctors make the difference between
life and death in the hospital. In reality, while the interns and residents that you see
in the hospital are doing their best, they are more likely to look like young versions
of Quincy than they are to solve medical mysteries like Quincy. In the real world, most
diseases and illnesses do not present as clearly as they do on television, and the
physicians have to make educated guesses about how to treat. In fact, if you had to
choose a hospital to take care of you or a loved one that had a reputation for great
physician care or great nursing care, you would be better off choosing the hospital
with great nursing care.

Why? There is a growing body of research that confirms a strong association between nursing care (e.g., staffing ratios, skill mix) and patient outcomes including morbidity and mortality (Nicklin & Graves, 2005). Simply put, patients in hospitals that are staffed by highly skilled nurses at sensible patient-to-nurse ratios (about four patients per nurse on a day shift) recover faster and live longer than their counterparts in hospitals with higher patient-to-nurse ratios (McCloskey & Diers, 2005; Rothberg, Abraham, Lindenauer, & Rose, 2005).

Sidebar 1-1

The Difference Between Nursing and Medicine

The focus of medicine is on disease. The physician wants to diagnose and treat disease. The focus of nursing is on the person rather than the disease. The nurse wants to figure out how a person lives (e.g., how they work, how they enjoy themselves, how they love) and how the disease affects how a person lives and what can be done about it.

Randolph Rasch, PhD, RN
Professor and Director of the Family Nurse Practitioner Specialty Vanderbilt University School of Nursing

---

I Don't Want Physicians Ordering Me Around

This is a concern that I have also heard many individuals express and relates to the perception that in the healthcare system physicians lord over nurses. I think television also contributes to this perception. On television (and in movies) the female nurse often acts as an unquestioning auxiliary to the male physician. In reality, nursing roles vary and some nurses collaborate better with physicians and other health disciplines than others. In hospitals, physicians and other licensed prescribing practitioners "write orders" for a medication or treatment that they want the nurse to administer. However, all registered nurses are bound by their licenses to carefully decide whether it is appropriate, or within their scope of practice, to administer this medication or treatment.

What is meant by "within their scope of practice"? Each state has a Nursing Practice Act (NPA) that defines the scope of practice or what activities a registered nurse may perform in that state. Individual state legislatures establish the content of the NPA, so NPAs are not exactly the same in every state; however, the NPAs address important issues defining the practice of nursing within that state. As Joel (2003) points out, the NPAs in each state contain the following basic components:

- Legislative mandate
- Definition of nursing

- Requirements for licensure
- Exemption from licensure
- Grounds for revocation
- Suspension or conditioning of the license
- Provision for endorsement for persons licensed in other states
- Creation of a board of nurse examiners
- Responsibilities of the board
- Penalties for practicing in violation of the act or without a license (p. 464).

Below is the NPA for New Jersey:

> The practice of nursing as a registered professional nurse is defined as diagnosing and treating human responses to actual or potential physical and emotional health problems, through such services as casefinding, health teaching, health counseling, and provision of care supportive to or restorative of life and well-being, and executing medical regimens as prescribed by a licensed or otherwise legally authorized physician or dentist. Diagnosing in the context of nursing practice means the identification of and discrimination between physical and psychosocial signs and symptoms essential to effective execution and management of the nursing regimen within the scope of practice of the registered professional nurse. Such diagnostic privilege is distinct from a medical diagnosis. Treating means selection and performance of those therapeutic measures essential to the effective management and execution of the nursing regimen. Human responses means those signs, symptoms, and processes which denote the individual's health need or reaction to an actual or potential health problem.

As stated in New Jersey's NPA, it is within the scope of nursing practice to execute medical regimens from other licensed providers; however, this statement makes it clear that the registered nurse must be selective in executing medical regimens "essential to the effective management and execution of the nursing regimen." This is a heavy responsibility and means that if nurses give a medication or apply a treatment that harms a patient, they are not protected by the fact that they were following orders. Nurses have to know what activities are within their scope of practice. To emphasize this point, the board of nursing in New Jersey provided a six-step algorithm to help nurses in deciding whether an activity is within their scope of practice:

1. Is the act consistent with your scope of practice in the New Jersey Nursing Practice Act? Do the Board's regulations address this specific act? If *no*, the

act is *not* within your scope of practice without the above. If *yes*, continue to the next step.

2. Is the activity authorized by a valid order, and in accordance with established institutional/agency or provider protocols, policies, and procedures? If *no*, the act is *not* within your scope of practice without the above. If *yes*, continue to the next step.

3. Is the act supported by research data from nursing literature and/or research from a health-related field? Has a national nursing organization issued a position statement on this practice? If *no*, the act is *not* within your scope of practice without the above. If *yes*, continue to the next step.

4. Do you possess the knowledge and clinical competence to perform this act safely? Documentation to validate your educational and clinical competence should be maintained for a 4-year period. If *no*, the act is *not* within your scope of practice without the above. If *yes*, continue to the next step.

5. Is the act to be performed within accepted "standards of care" that would be provided in similar circumstances by reasonable, prudent nurses with similar education and clinical skills? Nurses are accountable for knowing and conforming to their scope of practice in the NPA, board regulations, and any other state and federal laws affecting their practice. If *no*, the act is *not* within your scope of practice. Performance of the act may place the patient and the nurse at risk. If *yes*, continue to the next step.

6. Are you prepared to assume accountability for the provision of safe care? If *no*, the act is *not* within your scope of practice. If *yes*, you may perform the act based upon a valid order in accordance with the institution/agency or provider's established protocols, policies, and procedures.

As suggested by this algorithm, the NPAs broadly define what practices nurses may perform. The nurse's primary responsibility is to his or her patients (not physicians or hospital administrators), and nurses jeopardize their license if they engage in an activity that is not within their scope of practice.

Physicians Make More Than Nurses

I have spoken with many individuals who are interested in nursing but express a concern that, as compared to the salary of physicians, the nursing salary does not compare favorably. As one of these individuals put it, "It is not all about the money, but I can not act like money doesn't matter."

Physician Salary vs. Nurse Salary

So how much money do registered nurses make, and how much do physicians make? According to a 2006 report from the Bureau of Labor Statistics, the average hourly income for registered nurses is around $29 (Bureau of Labor Statistics, 2006). Of course, this is the average hourly income and, depending on what part of the country you are practicing in, this income will vary. For example, the average starting salary for nurses in New Jersey is about $66,000 per year (Bureau of Labor Statistics). The average salary for physicians also varies widely by geographical location and specialty; however, the average general practice physician earns about $137,000 per year (Bureau of Labor Statistics). Although it is clear that physicians make more in salary, there are some other factors that should be considered in comparing compensation.

Comparing Physician and Nurse Salaries

Cost of Education
First, the cost in terms of time and money of educating physicians is much greater than the cost of nursing education. In addition to completing 4 years of undergraduate education and 4 years of medical school, the typical physician also has a residency of 2 to 3 years. It makes sense that physicians should be compensated for the skills and knowledge that they have gained through this educational process.

Starting Work
Another factor that should be considered in comparing nursing salaries to physician salaries is that most physicians have to build up to making a six-figure salary. For most physicians the earliest age at which they would have completed their education is around 28 or 29, and during their residency period most physicians collect an annual salary that is well below six figures. For most nurses the earliest age at which they begin practicing full time as a nurse is around 22 years of age for graduates of baccalaureate programs (and earlier for graduates of diploma and associate degree programs). Consequently, a registered nurse who begins working full-time at 22 years

of age has the potential to have worked for at least 6 years before a physician begins earning near or at his or her potential.

Student Debt

In addition to entering the workforce later than most nurses, the average medical student accumulates more than $120,000 in debt by graduation (Kahn et al., 2006). Obviously, a debt of this size, even with a low-interest loan rate, eats up a substantial portion of one's income for many years. Consider that if we assume an interest of 7% on all combined loan debt and a repayment period of 10 years, the monthly payment on this loan is nearly $1,400. If we calculate that the average tax on annual income is about 30%, a physician earning $120,000 would bring home about $84,000 a year and $17,000 of that would go toward paying down the student loan debt. This leaves about $67,000.

Work Schedule

Another factor to consider is that most physicians and nurses who practice in the hospital do not work typical 9–5 hours. Many nurses work 12-hour shifts, and many physicians also work long hours that include evenings and weekends. One difference in job structure is that most nurses practicing in the hospital are usually paid for every hour they work, while physicians are more likely to work on a salary. Thus, if a nurse works overtime, he or she is paid for that additional time. In fact, according to data from the Bureau of Labor Statistics, nearly 30% of physicians reported that they worked more than 60 hours per week (Bureau of Labor Statistics, 2006). So it is true that physicians receive high pay, but they also work long hours. Based on the average salary for nurses and an overtime rate of salary plus 50%, a nurse working 60 hours per week can earn around $105,000 a year.

Nursing Is a Female Profession

Is nursing a female profession? Nursing is no more a female profession than race-car driving or engineering are male professions; however, while men are the predominant gender represented in those professions, women are the predominant gender in nursing, and it has become identified with the female gender. However, there are other factors that contribute to the perception that nursing is a female profession. Gender stereotypes contribute to this stereotypical perception. For example, as Meadus (2000) explained, the perception of women in nursing roles, "supports the stereotypical feminine image with traits of nurturing, caring, and gentleness in contrast to masculine characteristics of strength, aggression, and dominance" (p. 10).

There are also social and historical factors that have contributed to the female domination of nursing. For example, Florence Nightingale, known as the founder of modern nursing practice, promoted the image of nurses as nurturing, subordinate, and female (Meadus, 2000). And for a number of reasons this image took hold in society. One of the factors that solidified nursing as a female-dominated profession is that for most of the 1900s there were few professions open to women besides elementary school education, social work, and nursing and women are more likely to enter these fields for this reason.

However, the barriers that prevented women from entering other professions have pretty much eroded. The evidence that women are entering formely male-dominated fields is fairly strong. For example, there are an equal number of men and women applying to medical schools (Magrane & Jolly, 2002). It is estimated that by the year 2010, 40% of all attorneys will be women (Curran, 1995), and there are currently more female veterinarians than male veterinarians (Slater & Slater, 2000).

Although the proportion of women entering fields that were once male dominated has increased, the proportion of men entering the profession of nursing remains low. Why are so few men represented in the nursing field? Unfortunately, as reflected in the parenthetical statement, "I don't want to do women's work," there is evidence that some men are concerned that, because nursing is a female-dominated profession, a man who pursues a career in nursing is less manly (Boughn, 1994; Gray et al., 1996; Meadus, 2000; Williams, 1992). To dispel this misconception and increase the number of men in nursing, a number of media campaigns (e.g., calendars, posters) sponsored by groups supportive of nursing have sought to show men currently practicing as nurses who are nurses and also "manly" (e.g., men with black belts in karate, men who ride Harley motorcycles). In addition to these nursing-sponsored media campaigns, a growing number of television shows (e.g., *Scrubs*, *Heroes*) and movies (e.g., Ben Stiller's character in *Meet the Parents*) have featured more enlightened (and humorous) portrayals of men in nursing.

Even as most surveys estimate that men represent less than 6% of registered nurses, there is some evidence that these numbers may begin to change drastically in the near future (Health Resources and Services Administration, 2007). For example, the American Association of Colleges of Nursing (AACN) reported that 9% of nursing school students are men and, in some nursing schools, men account for greater than 25% of the students (Koloen, 2006). It is impossible to say whether this trend will continue; however, as more men enter nursing, it is difficult to imagine that nursing will continue to be characterized as "women's work." Moreover, as they say "nothing succeeds like success" and, while compensation and promotions are crude ways to measure success, by these measures men in nursing are more successful than their female counterparts. There is strong evidence that because of a variety of factors (e.g., higher levels of education, tendency to work intensive care jobs, no maternity leaves), men in nursing receive higher compensation and are more likely to be promoted into administrative positions than their female colleagues (Williams, 1992, 1995).

I Would Never Make It Through Nursing School

Many potential nursing school candidates fear the rigors of nursing school—and they should. I have told many students that all educational degrees are easy after nursing school. I have a nonnursing bachelor degree, a master's degree in nursing, and a PhD, and earning those degrees was not as challenging as earning my bachelor degree in nursing. What is so challenging about nursing school? Most people have a comfort zone, and I think the range of activities one has to engage in as a nursing school student pulls most individuals out of their comfort zone at one time or another. Few nurses will say that all aspects of nursing school were difficult; however, most nurses will be able to identify a certain aspect that was difficult for them. For example, some students struggle with the theoretical coursework but have no problem in the clinical setting, and for others the situation is reversed. For me, most aspects of clinical were easy but for some reason preparing medications was a steep challenge: I am a big picture thinker and sometimes important details like 25 mg or 2.5 mg get lost. For my wife, her psychiatric clinical rotation made her uncomfortable.

One of the keys to getting through nursing school lies in one's ability to put nursing school into the right perspective. An important component of this perspective is to focus on one's primary goal in nursing school. What is the goal of nursing school? Before answering that question, I will discuss what the goal of nursing school should *not* be. One's primary goal in nursing school should not be to survive it, or love it, or to get the highest grades in all of your classes. You are not studying nursing so that you can be a good nursing student any more than elementary school students are taught the alphabet so that they can sing the alphabet song with Big Bird and Elmo from *Sesame Street*. Children are taught the alphabet so that they can begin to learn to read.

One goes to nursing school to learn and develop the skills and knowledge one will need to become a competent and caring nurse. That is the purpose of nursing school. As a student and as a professor, I have known many students who have lost this focus and are more wrapped up in what they get as a score on a paper or an exam than what they learned. Educational psychologists such as Nicholls (1984) have argued that students who are engaged in this type of learning are ego-involved versus task-involved. Ego-involving situations are those where an individual's goal is to outperform others and where mastery of the task is a secondary goal; task-involving situations are those in which an individual's primary goal is to master the activity. There is strong evidence that students who focus on what they are learning rather than outperforming their peers or worrying what others think about them attain higher learning goals (Dweck, 2006; Graham & Golan, 1991; Nicholls, 1984).

I did not review any empirical evidence that suggests how common it is for nursing students to be ego-involved rather than task-involved; however, the anecdotal evidence suggests that it is too common. I have heard numerous faculty colleagues complain that students care only about their grades, and how they are tired of hearing students ask during a class: "Do I need to know this for the test?" or some question along those lines. You do not have to be the most empathetic person in the world to imagine that nursing faculty grow weary of hearing these types of questions. Consequently, not only does this type of ego-involved behavior diminish your learning, but posing these types of questions also degrades the learning environment.

The Physical and Mental Demands of Nursing School and Nursing

Providing excellent nursing care requires a great deal of physical and mental effort. Many nursing roles (e.g., hospital nursing, home care nursing) are done on one's feet—rather than sitting in front of a computer as I am now—and require the ability to perform some physical lifting. Moreover, nurses have to be able to critically process large amounts of information rapidly, prioritize needs, and take appropriate actions quickly. The minimum mental and physical qualifications laid out by the University of California, San Francisco, School of Nursing General Catalog (2007) include the following 11 requirements:

1. Lift and transfer patient up to 6 inches from a stooped position, then push or pull the weight up to 3 feet.
2. Lift and transfer patient from a stooped position to an upright position to accomplish bed-to-chair and chair-to-bed transfers.
3. Physically apply up to 10 pounds of pressure to bleeding sites or in performing cardiopulmonary resuscitation (CPR).

4.   Respond and react immediately to auditory impediments.
5.   Physically perform up to a 12-hour clinical laboratory experience.
6.   Perform close and distance visual activities involving objects, persons, and paperwork, as well as discriminate depth and color perception.
7.   Discriminate between sharp/dull and hot/cold when using hands.
8.   Perform mathematical calculation for medication preparation and administration.
9.   Communicate effectively, both orally and in writing, using appropriate grammar, vocabulary, and word usage.
10. Make appropriate and timely decisions under stressful situations.

As discussed, these requirements are minimal requirements for entry into a nursing program. Depending on one's career path after nursing school, the physical and mental requirements may be different.

Nurse's Reflection 1-1

I Never Wanted to Become a Nurse.
I Just Wanted a Free Dorm Room.

My older sister's agonizing experiences in a diploma school of nursing convinced me that I did not want to become a nurse, and I went to Queens College with the intention of becoming a math teacher or an architect. However, my career path changed when I wandered into the wrong room and heard the speaker tell the audience that students in the nursing program, "get a free dorm room in the city." At that moment I decided to become a nurse. It met my need to get away from home and still have free tuition and live in the middle of Manhattan. I do not know what I was thinking. I know I had no intention of eventually becoming a nurse. I just knew I needed to live in the city.

Off I went to Hunter College, living in the Bellevue School of Nursing dorms on 26 Street and First Avenue and commuting to liberal arts classes at 68th and Park. The first year required only one nursing course, lots of science, and mostly liberal arts. I continued into the heavy second year of medical surgical nursing, organic chemistry, and microbiology. Although it was not my cup of tea, I rationalized that I could not waste all of these credits so I would stay to see if there was another specialty I would like. As luck would have it, pediatrics and obstetrics were not for me either. I spent a good deal of time crying in pediatrics.

The next semester was the dreaded psychiatry. All of the upperclassmen warned us about the scary Bellevue tunnels and the giant key that got one in and out of the crazy ward. Students did not get a key, only the instructor. The patients were all said to be dangerous, and the wards were frightful. My interest was piqued! From day one, I loved the experience of psychiatric nursing. Despite all the tales, I found the patients responded if they knew you cared. I derived a great sense of accomplishment each day I spent there. I blossomed into the nurse I wanted to become through this clinical experience. This was the one area of nursing where I knew I excelled. It came with great ease, to listen to another and experience the world from another's perspective. I easily understood their acting out, their screams for help, their fears and paranoia. For 30 plus years I have spent my career working in mental health. I have derived great satisfaction by being present for others. My patients have each taught me more and more each day about what it means to care about another.

Sharon Kowalchuk, RN, MA
Instructor
Cochran School of Nursing

References

Boughn, S. (1994). Why do men choose nursing? *Nursing and Health Care, 15,* 406-411.

Bureau of Labor Statistics. (2006). Occupational Employment and Wages, May 2006. Retrieved March 21, 2008, from http://www.bls.gov/oes/current/oes291111.htm

Curran, B. A. (1995). *Women in the law: A look at the numbers.* Chicago: American Bar Association Commission on Women in the Profession.

Dweck, C. S. (2006). *Mindset: The new psychology of success.* Random House: New York.

Graham, S., & Golan, S. (1991). Motivational influences on cognition: Task involvement, ego involvement, and depth of information processing. *Journal of Educational Psychology, 83,* 187–194.

Gray, D. P., Kramer, M., Minick, P., McGehee, L., Thomas, D., & Greiner, D. (1996). Heterosexism in nursing education. *Journal of Nursing Education, 35,* 204–210.

Health Resources and Services Administration. (2007). *The registered nurse population: findings from the 2004 National Sample Survey of Registered Nurses.* Retrieved October 1, 2007, from http://bhpr.hrsa.gov/healthworkforce/rnsurvey04/3.htm

Joel, L. A. (2003). *Kelly's dimensions of professional nursing.* New York: McGraw-Hill.

Kahn, M. J., Markert, R. J. Lopez, F. A., Specter, S., Randall, H., & Krane, N. K. (2006). Is medical student choice of a primary care residency influenced by debt? *General Medicine, 8,* 100–112.

Koloen, J. (2006). More men heed the call to become nurses. *University of Texas Medical Branch Magazine.* Retrieved March 5, 2007, from http://www.utmb.edu/utmbmagazine/archive/06_ Spring/schoolnews/son/default.htm

Magrane, D., & Jolly, P. (2005) The changing representation of men and women in academic medicine. *Analysis in Brief, 5.* Retrieved February 7, 2007, from http://www.aamc.org/data/aib/ aibissues/aibvol5_no2.pdf

Marks, I. (1988). Blood-injury phobia: A review. *The American Journal of Psychiatry, 145*(10), 1207–1213.

McCloskey, B. A., & Diers, D. K. (2005). Effects of New Zealand's health reengineering on nurse and patient outcomes. *Medical Care, 43,* 1140–1146.

Meadus, R. (2000). Men in nursing: Barriers to recruitment. *Nursing Forum, 33,* 5–12.

Nicholls, J. (1984). Achievement motivation: Conceptions of ability, subjective experience, task choice, and performance. *Psychological Review, 91,* 328–346.

Nicklin, W., & Graves, E. (2005). Nursing and patient outcomes: It's time for healthcare leadership to respond. *Healthcare Management Forum, 18,* 40–45.

Rothberg, M. B., Abraham, I., Lindenauer, P. K., & Rose, D. N. (2005). Improving nurse-to-patient staffing ratios as a cost-effective safety intervention. *Medical Care, 43,* 785–791.

Slater, M. R., & Slater, M. (2000) Women in veterinary medicine. *Journal of the American Veterinarian Medical Association, 217,* 472–476.

University of San Francisco School of Nursing. (n.d.). *The University of San Francisco General Catalog 2007-2009.* Retrieved December 9, 2007, from http://www.usfca.edu/acadserv/ catalog/

Williams, C. L. (1992). The glass escalator. Hidden advantages for men in the "female" professions. *Social Problems, 29,* 253–268.

Williams, C. L. (1995). Hidden advantages for men in nursing. *Nursing Administration Quarterly, 19*(2), 63–70.

TWO

Who Is a Nurse, and How Does One Become a Nurse?

Who is a nurse? I recently heard the father of a US soldier who had been seriously wounded in Iraq interviewed on the radio. The father reported his son had received substandard care in a VA hospital. The father had been so dissatisfied with the care that his son received that he transferred his son to a private facility. During the interview, this father directed most of his anger and disappointment at "the nurses." He accused them of not doing their jobs and "let my son sit in human feces." As a father and an American citizen, I felt terrible for this man who only wanted the best care for his son, and as a nurse I felt a sense of shame that nurses were implicated. At the same time I could not help wondering who he was referring to when he said "nurses." Was he talking about certified nursing assistants, licensed practical nurses, registered nurses (RNs), nurse practitioners, advanced practice nurses? For most of the public, any woman in the hospital who is wearing anything that approximates a nursing uniform (e.g., scrubs) is a nurse. Resolving who is a nurse is beyond the scope of this book, but it is important to acknowledge that there is a great deal of confusion among the general public as to who is a nurse.

Pathways into Nursing

Part of this confusion stems from the fact that there is more than one pathway into nursing, and many people in the healthcare system are referred to as nurses. In this book, the title of nurse refers to RNs who have passed the National Council Licensure Examination (NCLEX). You can become eligible to take this exam through one of five ways, as shown in Figure 2-1.

Diploma Nursing School

Diploma nursing schools are often referred to as hospital schools of nursing because of their affiliation with hospitals. At one time, with few exceptions, this was the only way to receive educational preparation to become a nurse, and, in the early years, most nurses pursued no other formal education after receiving their diploma.[1] Joel (2003) reported that the proportion of total RNs who claimed the diploma as their highest educational credential declined from 63% in 1980 to 22.3% in 2000. For a variety of reasons the number of diploma nursing schools has declined significantly, and there are currently only 70 programs that offer a diploma in nursing (Bureau of Labor Statistics, 2006; Joel, 2003).

Associate Degree Programs

These programs are typically operated through junior colleges or community colleges and take about 2 years to complete. The number of associate degree (AD) programs has continued to grow steadily since the first three were introduced in 1952. As of 2006 there were about 850 AD nursing programs, and 40% of the current RN population received their initial nursing education in an AD program (American Nurses Association, 2008; Bureau of Labor Statistics, 2006; Joel, 2003).

Baccalaureate Nursing Programs

Most graduates of baccalaureate nursing programs receive a bachelor of science in nursing (BSN) (some baccalaureate programs confer a bachelor of arts), which takes

---

[1] Because most hospitals are not degree-conferring institutions, graduates of diploma schools can receive academic credit for their coursework only if the diploma school has developed a cooperative agreement with a college or university (Joel, 2003).

Figure 2-1   Five Pathways to Becoming a Registered Nurse

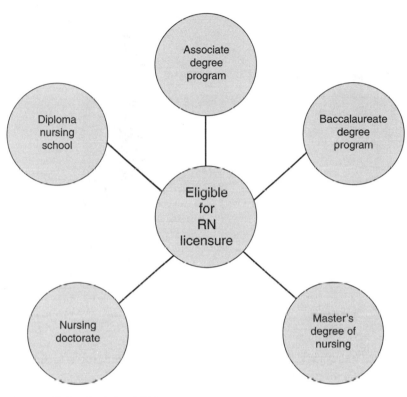

at least 4 years to complete. Of the total RN population in 2003, 29.3% held the baccalaureate as their initial preparation (Joel, 2003). According to the Bureau of Labor Statistics, in 2006 there were more than 706 BSN programs (Bureau of Labor Statistics, 2006).

Figure 2-2 is a bar graph depicting the number of nursing programs in the United States by program type. The graph was calculated based on data reported by the Bureau of Labor Statistics in 2006.

Other College/University Programs

Only a handful of institutions offer a master's degree of nursing (e.g., University of Minnesota) or the nursing doctorate (e.g., Case Western Reserve University) as the

Figure 2-2   Number of Nursing Programs by Type in the United States

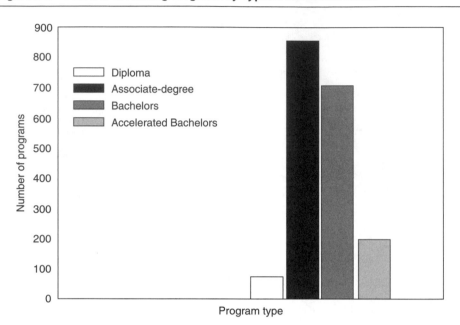

first professional degree; however, these programs are attractive to students who have already obtained one undergraduate degree.

Which Pathway into Nursing Is the Best?

Within the profession of nursing there is very strong feeling about the different pathways into nursing. One way to spark a debate among nurses is to say something like, "The best way to prepare nurses is through the _____ route" (insert one: diploma, associate, bachelor). In this debate, nurses educated in diploma and associate degree programs might argue that they had more clinical hours in their programs and came out of their programs more clinically prepared than their counterparts with bachelors. Bachelor-prepared nurses might argue that they got fewer clinical hours than their colleagues in diploma and associate degree programs, but their programs did a better job of preparing them to think critically and to assume leadership roles in nursing.

The best pathway into nursing for you will depend on a variety of factors such as your educational background, your career goals, and the programs that are available to you. For example, while I already had a bachelor degree when I began contemplating a career in nursing I pursued the baccalaureate route into nursing. This decision made the most sense for me for at least two reasons. First, I was living outside of Philadelphia, and there was an accelerated program for students who already had a baccalaureate degree in which the requirements for a BSN could be completed in less than two years. Second, I hoped to become a nurse practitioner, and I knew that most graduate programs in nursing required applicants to have a BSN.

Table 2-1 makes side-by-side comparisons for each of the pathways. The accelerated baccalaureate route has also been included.

Table 2-1 is only a general representation that applies to most students and most nursing programs, and, of course, there are exceptional circumstances or cases that are not accounted for by this table. For examples, students may take longer than 4 years to complete a baccalaureate program, graduates of diploma programs are not restricted to beginning their careers in hospital or acute-care settings, and some graduates of diploma programs may be able to skip the RN-BSN step and matriculate directly into a graduate program in nursing. As is often said in nursing, "It all depends," and Table 2-1 is just meant to provide a general reference point.

Advantages of Each Pathway

The advantages and disadvantages of each of pathway vary for each individual. For example, if an individual (let's call him Bart) is just graduating from high school, an advantage of the diploma and associate degree program for Bart might be that he could take a slightly quicker path to becoming an RN if he opted for a diploma or associate degree program rather than a baccalaureate route. In addition to becoming an RN in a shorter amount of time, Bart could start working as a nurse sooner than he would if he pursued the baccalaureate route, and there is the possibility that his employer might cover some or all of the tuition costs associated with obtaining a baccalaureate in nursing.

In contrast, if another student (let's call her Lisa) is what is referred to as a second-degree student (someone who has already received a bachelor degree), and if she is interested in becoming a nursing researcher, it would probably make more sense for her to pursue a baccalaureate degree in nursing. If Lisa is able to matriculate into one of the accelerated programs, she would probably be able to complete her program in about a year. Moreover, Lisa would have the educational preparation necessary to apply for admission to a doctoral program.

Table 2-1   Characteristics of Different Pathways to Becoming a Registered Nurse

	Diploma	Associate	Baccalaureate	Accelerated Baccalaureate Programs
Length of time to complete	2–3 years	1½ years to 3 years (as long as students have completed science and general education requirements)	4 years	1–1½ years
Admission requirements	• College preparatory coursework in high school	• College preparatory coursework in high school	• College preparatory coursework in high school • Scholastic Aptitude Test (SAT)	• Bachelor degree
Career starting point	• Employment in hospital or acute-care setting	• Employment in hospital or acute-care setting	• Employment in hospital or acute-care setting • Community practice • Ambulatory care centers	• Employment in hospital or acute-care setting • Community practice • Ambulatory care centers
Educational path	1. RN-BSN program 2. Graduate program	1. RN-BSN program 2. Graduate program	1. Graduate program	1. Graduate program

A Shameless Plug for Baccalaureate Preparation

Despite what I have written above regarding the advantages and disadvantages of the different nursing programs, I would be remiss if I did not mention that I advise all individuals interested in becoming RNs who do not have bachelor degrees to enroll in a baccalaureate program. In the interest of full disclosure, it should be noted that I received my nursing education in a baccalaureate program, and I currently teach in a baccalaureate program. However, my bias in favor of baccalaureate education for nurses goes beyond personal experiences.

There Is Value in a Liberal Arts Education

As Latzer (2004) emphasized in his study of higher education, a liberal arts education is valuable because (1) it provides a person with the analytical, writing, and quantitative skills needed to participate in our contemporary education; (2) it provides a person with the tools necessary to engage as a citizen; and (3) it allows a person to enjoy life-enriching elements of our civilization such as literature, philosophy, and music. The same values espoused by Latzer were stated almost two decades earlier in a pioneering document entitled *Essentials of College and University Education for Professional Practice* by the American Association of Colleges of Nursing (AACN) that proposed that graduates of baccalaureate programs in nursing be able to do all of the following:

1. Write, read, and speak English clearly and effectively to acquire knowledge, convey and discuss ideas, evaluate information, and think critically.
2. Think analytically and reason logically using verifiable information and past experience to select or create solutions to problems.
3. Understand a second language, at least at an elementary level, to widen access to the diversity of world culture.
4. Understand other cultural traditions to gain a perspective on personal values and the similarities and differences among individuals and groups.
5. Use mathematical concepts, interpret quantitative data, and use computers and other information technology to analyze problems and develop positions that depend on numbers and statistics.
6. Use concepts from the behavioral and biological sciences to understand oneself and one's relationship with other people and to comprehend the nature and function of communities.
7. Understand the physical world and its interrelationship with human activity to make decisions based on scientific evidence, and be responsive to the values and interests of the individual and society.

8.   Comprehend life and time from historical and contemporary perspectives, and draw from past experiences to influence the present and future.
9.   Gain a perspective on social, political, and economic issues for resolving societal and professional problems.
10. Comprehend the meaning of human spirituality to recognize the relationship of beliefs to culture, behavior, health, and healing.
11. Appreciate the role of the fine and performing arts in stimulating individual creativity, expressing personal feelings and emotions, and building a sense of the commonality of human experience.
12. Understand the nature of human values, and develop a personal philosophy to make ethical judgments in both personal and professional life.

As reflected in these 12 goals, a foundation in liberal arts increases the likelihood that a healthcare provider will be truly educated, compassionate, and socially conscious (Dellasega, Milone-Nuzzo, Curci, Ballard, & Kirch, 2007).

Real-World Snapshot 2-1

Understand the Big Picture of Your Nursing Education

Students should not sit passively and wait for the educational process to happen: they have the most important role in what they learn. Here are some recommendations to help students assume this role.

*   *Take the time to understand the plan of study at your nursing school.* Every nursing program has a plan of study for students that illustrates what students are expected to take and the sequence of those courses. This plan of study is not arbitrary, and it can give students a very clear understanding of what they are expected to know as they progress through the program.
*   *The humanities are part of nursing education for a reason.* Nursing is both an art and a science. That is one reason that most nursing students are required to take liberal arts and humanities courses such as literature and art history. If you are in an art appreciation class or a literature course, think about what you have learned in that course that you can take to your practice as a clinician. Think about how the artist sees the world and how it can inform your practice as a nurse. For example, if you go and look at a portrait exhibit, one

of the things that you should make note of is how that artist painted the skin. This is an important piece of clinical information because art imitates life, and artists pay close attention to the skin. As a nurse you have to be aware of the subtle coloration in the skin and think about: when are these colors within the norm and when are they abnormal? Even Matisse's portrait "The Green Line" (Madame Matisse, "The Green Line," 1905), which is a portrait of a woman with a green line down her nose, is an exaggeration but that color is in that face. One thing I do in the cultural diversity course that I teach is to encourage students to read literature and view cinema from other cultures. These kinds of activities give you a window into other cultures that is hard to get but is important to have in nursing because nurses need to understand the culture of others to provide culturally competent care.

- *Connect the dots in your education.* It is your responsibility to have a big picture and small picture perspective. Anything that you are taking should not be viewed as a waste of time. You should always be asking yourself: How is this course useful? How can I make this course useful? How does this new information fit with information that I learned in a previous course or courses?

Randolph Rasch, PhD, RN
Professor and Director of the Family Nurse Practitioner Specialty
Vanderbilt University School of Nursing

Better Patient Outcomes

There is a growing body of evidence that patients of baccalaureate-prepared nurses have better health outcomes. For example, in a study of Pennsylvania hospitals, Aiken and colleagues (2003) found that the proportion of BSN-prepared nurses was related to improved outcomes for surgical patients. As the proportion of BSN-prepared nurses on the nursing staff increased, so did the likelihood that providers responded to clinically important deteriorations that would have resulted in death and disability. In a study of Canadian hospitals, Tourangeau and colleagues (2007) showed an inverse association between the proportion of BSN-prepared nurses and the mortality rates of acute care patients. This means that as the proportion of BSN-prepared nurses on the nursing staff increases, the mortality rates decrease.

More study is needed to explain how and why patients in hospitals with higher proportions of BSN-prepared nurses do better than their counterparts in hospitals with lower ratios. However, it is reasonable to imagine that it may be partially attributable to educational differences between baccalaureate-prepared nurses and nurses from associate degree (AD) and diploma programs. For example, BSN programs are 1 to 2 years longer than AD and diploma programs and BSN students are required to take nursing leadership, community health nursing, and additional liberal arts and humanities courses as part of their preparation. Moreover, there are differences in the educational preparation of faculty at most BSN programs; faculty are frequently required to have a PhD as well as a master of science in nursing degree (Berlin & Sechrist, 2002). Without more study it is impossible to determine how these programmatic differences in education influence patient outcomes; however, there does seem to be a clear association between the educational preparation of nurses and patient outcomes. As Aiken and colleagues (2003) emphasized, nurses are the surveillance system in a hospital for errors and adverse occurrences, and it may be that BSN programs do a better job of preparing nurses to identify and respond to potential problems.

Equal Footing with Other Healthcare Professionals
My final reason for recommending that all nurses pursue a baccalaureate degree has to do with arguments made by nursing policy bodies, such as the American Nursing Association. The basic premise of these arguments is that nurses without a bachelor degree have less education than other healthcare workers such as physicians, occupational therapists, and social workers who all have at least a bachelor degree (and soon the entry level degree for occupational therapist, physical therapist, and pharmacists will be a clinical doctorate). As the argument goes, this disparity in education puts the nurses at a disadvantage when it comes to working effectively with these other healthcare professionals. While I think there is probably some merit to this argument, it should be noted that in my review of the literature I was unable to locate any strong evidence to support this argument. Moreover, there are likely to be a range of factors, other than education, that influence the working relationship between nurses and other healthcare professionals. These factors might include the structure of the healthcare institution, the personality of the nurse, the personality of the other healthcare professional, the work experience of the nurse, and so on.

References

Aiken, L. H., Clarke, S. P., Cheung, R. B., Sloane, D. M., & Silber, J. H. (2003). Educational levels of hospital nurses and surgical patient mortality. *Journal of the American Medical Association, 290,* 1617–1624.

American Nurses Association. (2008). Nursing education. Retrieved March 21, 2008, from http://nursingworld.org/EspeciallyForYou/StudentNurses/Education.aspx

Berlin, L. E., & Sechrist, K. R. (2002). The shortage of doctorally prepared nursing faculty: a dire situation. *Nursing Outlook, 50,* 50–56.

Bureau of Labor Statistics. (2006). Occupational Employment and Wages, May 2006. Retrieved March 21, 2008, from http://www.bls.gov/oes/current/oes291111.htm

Dellasega, C., Milone-Nuzzo, P., Curci, K. M., Ballard, J. O., & Kirch, D. G. (2007). The humanities interface of nursing and medicine. *Journal of Professional Nursing, 23,* 174–179.

Joel, L. A. (2003). *Kelly's dimensions of professional nursing.* New York: McGraw-Hill.

Latzer, B. (2004). *The hollow core. Failure of the general education curriculum. A fifty college study.* American Council of Trustees and Alumni. Retrieved September 12, 2007, from http://www.goacta.org/publications/Reports/TheHollowCore.pdf

Tourangeau, A. E., Doran, D. M., Hall, L. M., Pallas, L. O., Pringle, D., Tu, J. V., & Cranley, L. A. (2007). Impact of hospital nursing care on 30-day mortality for acute medical patients. *Journal of Advanced Nursing, 57,* 32–44.

THREE

What You Should Know About Nursing Faculty and the Structure of Nursing Programs

I have spent a great deal of time as a college student: I have two baccalaureate degrees, a master's degree, and a PhD. Despite spending so much time in institutions of higher learning, for most of my years as a college student I remained oblivious to how the system of education that I was investing so much time in was structured. I did not know or care about the motivations or pressures of the educators who taught my classes and clinicals and assigned my grades. I knew even less about the structure of the academic system. It was not until I started to get to the end of my doctoral studies that I began to take an interest in who my professors were professionally and how the academic structure they worked in functioned. I wished I had gained this information earlier in my academic career because I found that the academic process made more sense, and I got more out of it as I understood how it worked. In this chapter a discussion is provided on the priority of nursing programs, the motivations and pressures of faculty who teach in them, and the administrative organization of nursing schools.

Priorities of Nursing Schools

Approval by the State Board of Nursing

Nursing programs are typically based within institutions of higher education, such as universities or community colleges, or based within institutions like hospitals. No matter where the nursing program is based, administrators and faculty in all nursing schools have two fundamental priorities. The first is to be approved by the state board of nursing in their state. Without approval by the state board of nursing, a nursing program's graduates are ineligible to sit for the National Council Licensure Examination (NCLEX) and, in turn, cannot become registered nurses (RNs).

Accreditation

The other priority is to achieve and maintain accreditation. What is accreditation? Accreditation is a voluntary, self-regulatory process where nongovernmental organizations approve schools and programs that have been found to meet certain standards and criteria for educational quality. The two primary accrediting bodies for nurses are the National League for Nursing Accrediting Commission (NLNAC) and the Commission on Collegiate Nursing Education (CCNE). In the short term, accreditation is important because it permits students to take advantage of state and federal financial aid programs. In the long term, accreditation is important because many employers will only hire nurses from accredited programs, and students of programs without accreditation will have difficulty matriculating into RN-bachelor of science in nursing programs or graduate programs (Joel, 2003).

Accrediting agencies conduct in-depth reviews of programs that consider such questions as:

- How is the program structured? What are the qualifications of the faculty? What is in the curriculum?
- What are the rights and responsibilities of the students? How are students selected for admission?
- What resources does the program have to educate students? What are the clinical and community learning sites like?

To answer these questions, members of the accrediting agency look at performance on examinations (e.g., NCLEX); review documents (e.g., policies, curriculum documents, samples of tests, faculty qualifications); interview students, faculty, and administrators; and conduct on-site visits to classrooms and clinical sites (National Council of State Boards of Nursing, 2004).

NCLEX Pass Rate

As discussed above, the first-time pass rate of graduates on the licensure exam or the NCLEX is one standard by which nursing programs are evaluated. States vary slightly, but most states require that a nursing program has at least an 80% first-time pass rate of their graduates. A history of poor passing rates for first-time takers of the NCLEX-RN examination not only threatens accreditation but it also can impact a school's reputation, enrollment, and funding (Norton et al., 2006). Consequently, nursing programs invest a great deal of time into developing, implementing, and evaluating interventions designed to improve NCLEX passing rates (Beeson & Kissling, 2001; Daley, Kirkpatrick, Frazier, Chung, & Moser, 2003; Morrison, Free, & Newman, 2002; Seldomridge & DiBartolo, 2004).

The Faculty in Nursing Programs

As with most careers in nursing, nursing education has its own special set of challenges. The challenges and stressors experienced by the faculty members teaching in your nursing program have to do with the faculty members and your nursing program. For example, while there are some stressors that all educators feel (e.g., am I prepared to teach today?), a master's-prepared clinical instructor within a department of nursing at a community college probably has a different set of concerns than a doctorally prepared associate professor in a college of nursing at a major research university. Understanding the motivations (e.g., what makes a person tick) and the frustrations (e.g., what ticks a person off) of the educators in your nursing program will help you get the most out of the nursing school experience. Moreover, empathy, or an awareness of another individual's life challenges, is a trait common to most excellent nurses. In the sections that follow, discussion is provided that will help you gain a better understanding of the faculty member teaching in your nursing program.

Faculty Educational Background

Virtually all faculty teaching in diploma, associate, and baccalaureate degree programs, as well as administrators directing nursing programs, are required to hold at least a master's degree in nursing and to have clinical experience relevant to their clinical areas of responsibility. This means that a nursing faculty member who teaches pediatric theory or pediatric clinical will have experience working with children and families.

Many baccalaureate degree programs require that, in addition to a master's degree, faculty teaching in baccalaureate programs have either an earned doctorate or a specific plan for completing a doctorate. Most doctorally prepared nursing faculty with appointments at colleges and universities in the United States have doctorates that are considered terminal degrees or academic degrees of the highest level. This type of degree usually takes at least 3 years of full-time study following the completion of a master's degree, and a dissertation must be completed. These doctorates are the PhD, a doctor of education, or a doctor of nursing science. A growing number of nursing schools are offering doctor of nursing practice (DNP) programs that prepare nurses for clinical practice or clinical leadership. Although the DNP is an advanced-level degree, in nursing it is not a terminal degree.

Teaching and Clinical Teaching Responsibilities

All nursing faculty are expected to have knowledge of nursing and clinical expertise in the subject area in which they teach (Joel, 2003). In contrast to the content in other disciplines—such as statistics or English literature—the evidence that guides practice in nursing needs to be updated frequently, and all faculty have to stay current with this information to teach effectively.

In addition to the stress of staying current with clinical knowledge, many faculty members in nursing programs are burdened by the task of passing on that clinical knowledge and expertise to students through clinical teaching. The teaching responsibilities vary by educational institution and position; however, there is evidence that clinical teaching responsibilities are a common source of stress for most nursing faculty (Goldenberg & Waddell, 1990; Lott, Anderson, & Kenner, 1993; Oermann, 1998). While some faculty members in baccalaureate programs (e.g., tenure-track faculty) are not required to provide clinical or lab instruction, many faculty in diploma, associate, and baccalaureate programs are responsible for providing classroom, laboratory, and clinical instruction in their area of clinical expertise (e.g., medical/surgical, family, or psychiatric nursing). The burdens of clinical teaching are two-fold in that (1) the time required to provide clinical teaching is substantial (e.g., 6–8 hours per clinical day), and (2) faculty members must spend time in tasks related to clinical teaching such as making clinical assignments and reviewing nursing care plans submitted by students (Oermann, 1998).

Nonteaching Responsibilities

Regardless of the nursing program, all full-time faculty members also have responsibilities to contribute to the organization and functioning of the nursing program. Joel (2003) describes these varying committee responsibilities:

> Some are development and updating of philosophy, objectives, conceptual framework, and selecting appropriate courses to meet those objectives; selection, evaluation, and promotion of students; assisting in developing educational and faculty standards, policies, and procedures; participating in promotion and tenure of faculty; developing special projects; and planning for the future (p. 345).

These committee responsibilities require weekly and monthly meetings throughout the academic year and committee work that has to be completed independently of committee meetings. In addition to committee work, faculty in nursing programs are also required to make time available to advise and counsel students.

Concerns over Contractual Agreements and Appointments

Due to the severe nursing faculty shortage, fewer nursing faculty in diploma, associate, and baccalaureate degree programs are preoccupied with concerns of steady employment. However, this is not true for all faculty in baccalaureate nursing programs.

Faculty in Diploma and Associate Degree Nursing Programs

While there has been a substantial increase in the number of part-time and adjunct faculty in diploma, associate, and baccalaureate nursing programs, most faculty in diploma and associate degree programs have contractual agreements that can be renewed on a semester-by-semester basis or a yearly basis. Depending on the program, nursing educators with these roles within the institution may be classified as full-time or part-time employees.

Faculty in Baccalaureate Degree Nursing Programs

Nursing educators who are employed in nursing programs within colleges or universities are usually appointed to clinical-track or tenure-track positions. Depending on their educational background and scholarly achievements, nursing faculty may be appointed to one of the following academic ranks:

- Instructor—Individuals who have successfully completed all requirements for the doctorate or terminal degree, but who have not yet successfully defended or otherwise attained the degree, may be appointed to this rank with the stated expectation that, upon completion of the degree, the faculty member will be appointed to the rank of assistant professor.
- Assistant professor—Exceptions are sometimes made; however, a doctorate or terminal degree is usually required for this rank. This is usually the first academic rank for nursing faculty.
- Associate professor—In addition to the requirements for assistant professor, an individual with this rank must demonstrate good to excellent teaching performance. The candidate should be engaged in scholarship, research, or other creative activities and university service that are likely to result in additional academic achievements.
- Professor—Appointment to this rank is usually reserved for individuals who have achieved national recognition for their academic achievements as a scholar, teacher, or leader in the field of nursing.

Faculty who have clinical-track appointments—appointments in which clinical practice rather than scholarship is the primary criterion for promotion—or who have appointments as lecturers and assistant professors usually receive contracts of employment ranging from 1 to 3 years. In contrast, at most colleges and universities the associate professor and professor faculty have what is known as tenure.

The Tenure Process

Most colleges and universities in the United States and Canada have a system that allows faculty at that institution to achieve lifetime tenure or a contractual right not to be fired. Why have colleges and universities adopted a tenure system? The primary reason for tenure is to protect the freedom of faculty to honestly express opinions and ideas or engage in activities that might be controversial. Of course, there are cases in which tenure can be withdrawn, such as being convicted of a felony or gross incompetence; however, the revocation of tenure is rare. Less than 75 tenured professors out of 280,000 in the United States lose their positions for cause each year (Lublin, 2005). Another benefit of tenure is that, as you might guess, it is an extremely attractive job benefit that lures many into academia.

To achieve tenure at most institutions, nursing faculty have to demonstrate significant accomplishments in the following areas:

- Grant funding—An expectation of nursing faculty at most universities is that they will attract external funding to support their research activities. This external funding can come in the form of private funding from foundations such as the Robert Wood Johnson Foundation or federal funding from agencies such as the National Institutes of Health. The amount of grant funding that is considered sufficient for tenure depends on a number of factors, including the other accomplishments of the faculty and the university.

- Scholarship—In addition to grant funding, another expectation of tenure-track nursing faculty is that they engage in scholarship that contributes to knowledge in nursing and health. Nursing faculty typically demonstrate their scholarly worth by conducting studies (usually financed through grant funding discussed above) and then disseminating the findings of their studies by authoring journal articles that appear in refereed publications. To have an article appear in a refereed publication, the author must submit a manuscript to a journal where an editor calls on experts in the field to review the manuscript. The reviewers make recommendations as to whether the manuscript is likely to contribute to the field of nursing and health, and they provide feedback to the author on ways to improve the manuscript. Based on this review process, a decision is made by the journal editor to publish the manuscript, to have the author revise and resubmit the manuscript, or to reject the manuscript for publication in that journal.

- Teaching—An expectation of all faculty is that they be effective teachers in the classroom and in clinical practice. A faculty member's effectiveness as a teacher is assessed through peer evaluations and student evaluations. It is worth noting that, in contrast to your high school and elementary school teachers, your teachers in nursing school have little if any formal training in education. Most faculty have to figure out how to be effective in the classroom through trial and error.

- Service—In addition to teaching, scholarship, and the pursuit of grant funding, faculty on the tenure track are also expected to contribute to their department, the university, their profession, and society at large through service. This service involves participation on departmental committees and university committees to improve student academic development, participation on editorial boards as reviewers, and contributions to the common good by providing public service in their local, state, and national communities.

In most institutions failure to attain tenure results in the tenure candidate being dismissed from that institution. Faculty members are like most other employees in that they do not want to be forced to leave their job and seek other employment, relocate, and possibly begin the whole tenure process at another institution. Consequently, the pressures to attain tenure can be a source of great stress for faculty members in all academic disciplines. In a study of 100 baccalaureate nursing faculty, Melland (1995) found that the majority of participants perceived the pressure to publish to be high. Moreover, there is some evidence that the clinical teaching load and faculty practice requirements may diminish the likelihood that nursing faculty will attain tenure (Balogun, Sloan & Germain, 2006; Eddy, 2007).

Administration

In addition to the faculty, nursing programs often have a range of administrators and administrative staff. The lead administrator in any nursing program is the chair of the department or, in a school or college of nursing, the dean. In a nursing department, the chair's responsibilities typically include supervising the professional staff of faculty and administrative assistants, preparing annual performance evaluations, maintaining records and budget, scheduling classes and assigning teaching loads, and maintaining and revising curricula. The responsibilities of a dean in a college or school of nursing include some of the chair responsibilities but also include developing and implementing a vision for the college or school of nursing. The dean usually reports directly to the top academic administrator within the university.

Depending on the size of the nursing program, there may be several other administrators who report to the chair or dean. In a large school or college of nursing, these administrators have titles of associate or assistant deans. Figure 3-1 represents the organizational structure for a diploma/associate degree program and a baccalaureate program within a school of nursing at a college or university. As you would expect, the organizational chart for the baccalaureate program is more complex because these programs tend to be larger with a greater number of faculty members, administrators, and administrative staff.

Figure 3-1   Organizational Structure for a Diploma/Associate Degree Program and a Baccalaureate Program Within a School of Nursing at a College or University

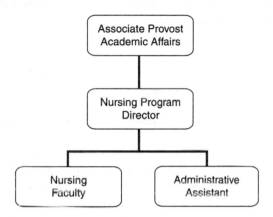

Figure 3-1a   Diploma/Associate Degree Program

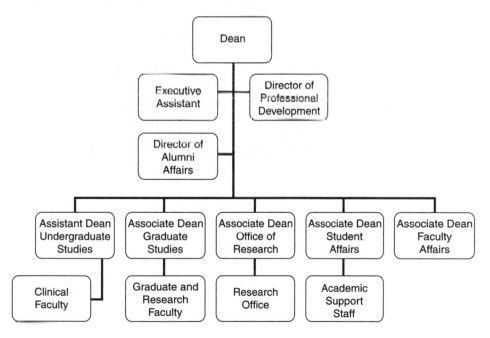

Figure 3-1b   Baccalaureate Program Within a School of Nursing at a College or University

References

Balogun, J. A., Sloan, P. E., & Germain, M. (2006). Determinants of tenure in allied health and nursing education. *Journal of Advanced Nursing, 56,* 532–541.

Beeson, S. A., & Kissling, G. (2001). Predicting success for baccalaureate graduates on the NCLEX-RN. *Journal of Professional Nursing, 17,* 121–127.

Daley, L. K., Kirkpatrick, B. L., Frazier, S. K., Chung, M. L., & Moser, D. K. (2003). Predictors of NCLEX-RN success in a baccalaureate nursing program as a foundation for remediation. *Journal of Nursing Education, 42,* 390–398.

Eddy, L. L. (2007). Evaluation research as academic scholarship. *Nursing Education Perspectives, 28,* 77–81.

Goldenberg, D., & Waddell, J. (1990). Occupational stress and coping strategies among female baccalaureate nursing faculty. *Journal of Advanced Nursing, 15,* 531–543.

Joel, L. A. (2003). *Kelly's dimensions of professional nursing.* New York: McGraw-Hill.

Lott, J. W., Anderson, E. R., & Kenner, C. (1993). Role stress and strain among nondoctorally prepared undergraduate faculty in a school of nursing with a doctoral program. *Journal of Professional Nursing, 9,* 14–22.

Lublin, J. (2005, January 10). Travel expenses prompt Yale to force out institute chief. *Wall Street Journal.* p. B1.

Melland, H. I. (1995). Nurse educators and the demands of research. *Journal of Nursing Education, 34,* 71–76.

Morrison, S., Free, K., & Newman, M. (2002). Do progressions and remediation policies improve NCLEX-RN pass rates? *Nurse Educator, 27,* 94–96.

National Council of State Boards of Nursing. (2004). White paper on the state of the art of approval/accreditation processes in boards of nursing. Retrieved August 1, 2007, from https://www.ncsbn.org/Final_11_05_Approval_White_Paper.pdf

Norton, C. K., Relf, M. V., Cox, C. W., Farley, J., Lachat, M., Tucker, M., & Murray, J. (2006). Ensuring NCLEX-RN success for first-time test takers. *Journal of Professional Nursing, 22,* 322–326.

Oermann, M. H. (1998). Work-related stress of clinical nursing. *Journal of Nursing Education, 37,* 302–304.

Seldomridge, L. A., & DiBartolo, M. C. (2004). Can success and failure be predicted for baccalaureate graduates on the computerized NCLEX-RN? *Journal of Professional Nursing, 20,* 361–368.

FOUR

Getting into Nursing School

As discussed earlier, there are not enough nurses to meet the current or future healthcare demands in this country. One factor influencing this shortage is that, while more individuals are applying to nursing school than ever before, nursing schools are unable to admit many qualified applicants because there are not enough educators to teach them nor are there enough clinical sites to train nurses. How many qualified applicants are being denied admission to nursing school? One study found that in 2005 more than 41,000 qualified applicants were denied admission to nursing school (PricewaterhouseCoopers, 2007). This finding is consistent with the conversations I have had with many nursing school administrators and faculty who complain that they are turning away or wait-listing tremendous applicants—candidates with GPAs near 4.0, great letters of reference, well-written personal essays—because they do not have the capacity to admit these students.

The focus of this book is on providing guidance on how to make the most of your nursing school education and your early career in nursing. Of course, this guidance is not worth very much if you are unable to get into nursing school. The focus of this chapter is on how to improve your chances of being admitted into nursing school.

What Are Nursing Schools Looking for in Applicants?

Strong Academic Background

As discussed, the course and clinical requirements in nursing are challenging, the cost of educating nurses is high, and there are more students interested in going to nursing school than spots available within nursing schools; consequently, nursing schools have good reason to select the applicants who stand the best chance of being successful in nursing school and passing the National Council Licensure Examination (NCLEX). Moreover, nursing schools want to select students who will make meaningful contributions to society as nurses and citizens. How do nursing schools choose these individuals? It is unlikely to come as a surprise that nursing schools want to enroll students with strong academic backgrounds. Students who have demonstrated high levels of academic achievement in other contexts (e.g., high school, previous undergraduate coursework) are likely to be successful in nursing school. Nursing schools are especially interested in identifying students who are strong in math and sciences because there is some evidence that these students are more successful in nursing school and more likely to pass the NCLEX on the first attempt (Yin & Burger, 2003).

Baccalaureate Nursing Programs

Baccalaureate nursing programs vary in how they admit applicants. Some baccalaureate programs admit applicants in their first year. For example, at Rutgers, the State University of New Jersey, where I am a faculty member, applicants may be admitted directly into the College of Nursing. Admission into these programs is competitive and typically based on high school GPA and SAT scores. Baccalaureate programs also admit applicants as transfer students or accelerated students (students who received a bachelor degree in another major). Admission as a transfer or accelerated student to these programs is also competitive; however, committees evaluating these applicants typically have more criteria on which to evaluate applicants. In addition to SAT scores and high school GPA, the committees can also look at undergraduate GPAs with an emphasis on the sciences (microbiology, anatomy, physiology, and chemistry).

Associate and Diploma Nursing Programs

In evaluating the academic fitness of applicants to these programs, admission committees typically focus on high school GPA and the prerequisite science courses. A growing number of associate and diploma nursing programs have also begun using entrance exams. The most popular of these entrance exams is the Nurse Entrance Test (NET) that assesses basic math skills, science, reading comprehension, and learning styles. There is some evidence that scores on the NET exam are predictive of nursing school success (Sayles, Shelton, & Powell, 2003).

In sum, the demand for admission into nursing school is much greater than the supply of slots in nursing school. There is some evidence to indicate that there is some predictability to success in nursing school and the all-important NCLEX exam. In most cases nursing programs weigh these predictors heavily in their admission decisions. Applicants to nursing school who have strong reading and math skills, above average scores on standardized tests, and high GPAs are considered "safer bets" than their counterparts who have not performed as well, and, in turn, these "safer bets" are more likely to be admitted to nursing school.

Person-Based Qualities

Although academic ability and classroom-based qualities are important and weighed heavily by nursing school admission committees, they are not (and should not be) the only determinant of who gets into nursing school and becomes a nurse. The challenges of nursing are substantial and require more than the ability to do well in the classroom. There are a number of person-based qualities that nurses need to have. Leners, Beardslee, and Peters (1996) developed a list of additional *relevant assets* that nursing school admission committees should consider in applicants. This list includes the following five person-based qualities:

Sidebar 4-1

Recommendation for Prospective Students Who Are Parents of Infants or Young Children

Ask yourself is this the right time to go back to school? The first thing I tell prospective students who are parents of very young children, especially those parents without extensive support networks, is that it may not be the right time to go back to school. If the kids are in school or daycare all day and the student is able to carve out a solid block of uninterrupted time a couple of days a week when they can study, practice test questions, and meet with their professors if they need to, then they have a shot at being a successful student. The uninterrupted block of time during the week is crucial. Weekends are not enough because the kids are usually home, and students have to parent. Similarly, staying up late at night and trying to cram is not going to work either because the nursing student becomes sleep deprived.

Jane Kurz, PhD, RN
Associate Professor
Department of Nursing, Temple University

1. Ability to communicate effectively
2. Self-awareness and an understanding of the effect of the self on others
3. Identification of personal gifts and talents with creative application of the same to nursing practice
4. Ability to solve problems and the ability to reflect on life experiences
5. Awareness of healthcare issues as they affect nursing; and understanding of nursing as a professional career (p. 138).

Measures such as your GPA and scores on standardized tests do not tell the whole story of who you are and your potential to be successful in nursing school and in nursing. One of your goals in developing your application to nursing school is to show admission committees the person-based qualities that you have in addition to your academic abilities. Discussed in this section are suggestions on how to showcase your person-based qualities in your application.

The Application Process

The Personal Statement

The personal statement (which is usually an essay but sometimes a letter) is an important component in the application of all nursing school applicants. For applicants with strong academic backgrounds, the personal statement provides an opportunity to show that they are more than good students. For applicants with shaky academic backgrounds, it provides an opportunity to show that they have personal strengths that make them good nursing school candidates. In either case you want to make the most of the personal essay to showcase yourself. The first step in writing a strong personal essay is to give yourself enough time to get your thoughts together about how you decided to become a nurse and what you want to do as a nurse. Leners and colleagues (1996) proposed three themes that can be used to focus your thinking:

1. Describe talents, aptitudes, or gifts you possess and show how these could contribute to a nursing career (e.g., art, music, computer literacy).
2. Describe any life experiences that have contributed to your interest in nursing as a career (e.g., leadership roles, community service).
3. Describe how you envision yourself, as a nurse, practicing in the United States healthcare system in the next 5 years.

In addition to writing personal essays that incorporate these themes, there are a number of well-written guides on the subject of writing essays and personal statements for admission to undergraduate and graduate programs. I have adapted some of the recommendations included in Richard Stelzer's (1989) book *How to Write a Winning Personal Statement for Graduate and Professional School* for this section.

Answer the Questions That Are Asked

Nurses have to be good communicators, and part of good communication involves answering questions that are asked of you. If you are applying to more than one nursing school, it is likely that you may get questions for personal statements that are similar. Do not give in to the temptation to submit the same personal statement for each application to avoid having to write another personal statement. Push yourself to develop an individual statement that will make sense to the reviewers by crafting a personal statement that relates to the questions that are asked.

Tell a Story

Admission committee members read numerous personal statements, and all of them start to look the same after the first few. You want your personal statement to grab the reader's attention and stand out from the rest. After reading your personal statement, the reader should think, "This would be an interesting person to have on campus or in a class." One way to get this reaction is to tell a story in your personal statement. Most people would rather read a story than a traditional five-paragraph essay, and you do not have to be Stephen King or J. K. Rowling to make a story out of why you want to be a nurse or what you want to do as a nurse. For example, if you were hospitalized as a child or adolescent and that experience motivated you to become a nurse, use specific details (e.g., the beep of the monitor, the smell of the hospital) of the experience to show the reader what you experienced and how you came to know nurses during that hospital stay.

Find an Angle

Make sure the details that you include in your personal statement are memorable or distinctive. For example, if you were hospitalized as a child because you were struck by lightning or were attacked by a swarm of bees, make sure to be expansive in your discussion of this experience. Few people have had these types of experiences, and you may stick in the memory of the admission committee as the "lightning guy" or "killer-bee fighter."

Focus on Your Opening Paragraph

As discussed, the admission committees read numerous personal statements, and you want your statement to be read with interest, so focus on writing a great first paragraph. You want to give the reader the idea of what you are going to share in your personal statement and you want to make it clear that what you are going to include is something very interesting, if not spectacular.

Show What You Know

You want to show, rather than tell, the reader what happened or what you know about nursing in your personal statement as much as possible. Consequently, if volunteering at a nursing home or taking care of your brother with special needs sparked your interest in nursing, make sure you include some details of what you learned in those roles. Discuss what you know about medications, Medicare reimbursement, or taking a blood pressure reading from experiences, classes, conversations with healthcare professionals, or books you have read. Use the terminology and language of the nursing profession to show the reader that you did not just wake up one morning and decide that you wanted to become a nurse.

Do Your Research

Maybe you did just wake up one morning and decide that you wanted to become a nurse. If this is the case, get a better understanding of nursing by doing some research of your own. This type of research might include talking to as many nurses as possible in different specialties about nursing, reading some nursing journals and books such as this one, and spending a day with a nurse if possible. Moreover, do some research on the institution that you are applying to and think about why this institution would help you meet your professional goals. For example, if you are applying to a nursing school at a research university, look at the faculty Web pages and make note of faculty who are doing research that you find interesting. For example, a professor may be conducting research on improving the health of babies born prematurely, and you may have an interest in this topic. In your personal statement discuss how your interests intersect with the research interests of the faculty and how that influenced your decision to apply to that institution.

Avoid Controversy

While you want your personal statement to stand out, you do not want it to stand out because you have discussed some controversial religious or political matter in your personal statement. To thine own self be true, but avoid topics (e.g., abortion, legalization of marijuana, death penalty) that may offend the readers of your personal statement, if at all possible. Moreover, make sure you know where you are applying and think about the reviewers. For example, if you are applying to a nursing program that is affiliated with the Catholic church, you probably do not want to submit a personal statement emphasizing how you want to become a nurse so that you can work in a family planning clinic.

Pay Attention to Your Writing

Nobody wants to read personal statements that have grammatical and spelling errors, incorrect use of language, and poorly constructed sentences. Spelling and grammatical errors are especially irksome for admission committees because of the availability of word-processing programs that identify errors. Make sure that your personal statement has been thoroughly proofread by you and at least two others that you trust (having your younger brother in the 8th grade as a reader is probably not going to help your cause). You want your personal statement to read well and to be error free. These goals will be difficult to achieve if you do not begin working on your personal statement well ahead of the deadline, so do not procrastinate. (See Appendix 4-A and Appendix 4-B for a sample admissions essay with a critique and a sample letter with a critique.)

The Interview

The personal interview is usually not required (and for some schools of nursing not an option); however, if you have the opportunity to interview with an alumnus, admissions officer, or student of an institution you are applying to, you may want to consider scheduling an interview. Like your personal statement, the interview adds another dimension to your application packet and, unless you do something wildly inappropriate (e.g., show up for your interview wearing a batman costume), the interview will only enhance your chances of admission. Unlike all of the other documents in your application packet, the interview allows someone other than you and those you trust (your references) to represent you to the admissions committee. The interview is also a chance for you to ask questions about the institution to which you are applying.

Most people will be anxious about a personal interview—this is normal. Although there is evidence that a certain level of anxiety may contribute to improving your performance, overwhelming anxiety is no good. There are a few things that you can do to lessen your anxiety about an interview. First, put the interview in perspective. As noted, unless you do something inappropriate, the interview will only enhance your chances of admission.

Second, prepare yourself for the interview. There are a finite number of questions that an interviewer is likely to ask you during an interview; if you practice answering

these questions during mock interview sessions, you will have the chance to formu-
late thoughtful responses and practice answering questions. Moreover, you will diminish some of your anxiety. Practice answering such questions with friends or
family members.

Sidebar 4-2

Interview Questions

Why do you want to attend *X*
    university?
What is your strongest point?
    Weakest point?
What have you done to
    prepare for college?
What has been your greatest
    experience in high school?
What do you want to do in
    the future?
Tell me about yourself (focus
    on about three things).
Tell me about your interests.
Tell me about your
    involvement in
    extracurricular activities.
Tell me about your family.
What do you think about
    (insert a current event of
    the past week)?
What is your favorite book?
    Who is your favorite author?
Which of your
    accomplishments are you
    most proud of?
If you could meet any
    important figure in the past
    or present, who would it be
    and what would you talk
    about?

Source: Tanabe and Tanabe, 2007.

Letters of Recommendation

Most nursing schools also require at least two letters of recommendation from individuals who
were your mentors, educators, or supervisors. You
should be thoughtful and strategic in whom you
ask to complete the recommendation forms because admission committees use them to get a fix
on the person-based qualities that you possess
and the likelihood that you will do well in nursing school and contribute to the profession of
nursing. Think it through before you give someone a letter of recommendation to submit on your
behalf. Ask yourself: "Have I done anything to
turn this person against me?" (e.g., got him au-
dited by the IRS, forgot to let her dog out while
she was on vacation). You do not want to be the
otherwise strong applicant who received only
marginally positive recommendations ("damned
with faint praise") and denied admission to
nursing school while another applicant who was
not as strong as you academically, but received
glowing recommendations, gained acceptance to
nursing school.

You want to choose individuals who can provide you with a glowing recommendation. In the
discussion that follows, recommendations are provided on how to improve the prospects that your
recommendations put you in the best light and improve the likelihood that you will be admitted to
nursing school.

Make Sure That Your Reference Knows You

The first section of the recommendation form asks the individual filling out the form to indicate how long that individual has known you and in what capacity. In choosing a person to write you a letter of reference, you have to be selective and find someone with whom you have some history. The teacher that you had for only a half of a semester or your work supervisor who was just hired and calls you by the wrong name most of the time is not who you want to ask to provide a letter of recommendation. Look carefully at the recommendation form and what needs to be filled out in deciding on who knows you well enough and in what capacity to provide a letter of recommendation. You want a reference who is able to assess you on at least 75% of the categories and questions.

Make Sure That They Like You

In addition to assessing you in at least three quarters of the categories, you want a reference who will have good things to say about you. The second section of most recommendation forms asks references to rate personal qualities of applicants such as critical thinking, character, resourcefulness, and reliability. The references rate applicants' personal qualities from 1 (Excellent) to 5 (Poor). You should not assume that just because you ask someone to serve as a reference they will evaluate you favorably. In fact, there is nothing wrong with asking a potential reference whether he or she will be able to provide you with a strongly favorable recommendation.

Choose Someone Who Will Meet the Deadline

Another factor to consider in choosing a reference is choosing someone who is responsible and able to meet a deadline. If recommendation forms are not mailed in by the deadline, there is the possibility that your application will not be reviewed. A great reference does you no good if it does not get read, so find someone who is reliable and orderly. In addition, most recommendation forms are mailed back to the applicant or submitted online. Make sure that you give the recommendation form or submission information to your reference well ahead of the deadline and that you provide a self-addressed stamped envelope to the reference if the form needs to be mailed.

Help Out the Reference

You can also make the process easier for your reference by providing information that may help the reference write about you. This information will assist the reference in completing the final section of most recommendation forms. This final section requires the reference to answer questions about your personal qualities by providing specific examples. A page or two of information about yourself will make the process of answering these questions much simpler for your reference and make the reference letter more descriptive. Information that you might consider giving to your reference is often termed a *biographical sketch*. This short narrative statement provides your reference with some information on the educational, work, or personal experiences that you have had that could contribute to your nursing career. You could also give your reference a resume and a draft of the personal statement that you are submitting with your application. This will allow the reference to write something that fits with the story or theme you have developed in your personal statement.

How to Handle Being Denied Admission to Nursing School

As discussed above, a number of qualified applicants are not being admitted into nursing school. Following the suggestions discussed in this chapter will improve your likelihood of being admitted to nursing school; however, you may be one of the qualified applicants denied admission. Discussed in this section are suggestions for what to do to improve your chances of being admitted to nursing school in the future.

Take Some Time to Cool Off

Although you may understand that competition for admission into nursing school is very stiff, it is hard not to get one's hopes up for admission and even harder not to be disappointed when your hopes are not fulfilled. As an assistant professor, I spend a substantial amount of time writing research funding proposals to different private and federal funding agencies, and while I understand that funding is limited, it always wounds my ego when a proposal is denied funding. I have all sorts of self-doubt and second thoughts about whether I am cut out to do research, and I wonder if I should switch careers. I also have angry thoughts, and a part of me wants to pick up the phone and call the review committee members and tell them that they are idiots. Fortunately, I have learned that it is best not to make any life-changing decisions or burn any bridges within 24 hours of receiving a wound to my ego. In the 24 hours after receiving bad news, I share my thoughts with people who love me, I exercise, I get a good·night's sleep, and I play with my kids. These actions give me time to cool off and get some perspective. If you are denied admission to nursing school, you should probably take more time (maybe several days) to cool off and get some perspective. If you are a qualified applicant and you have a strong desire to become a nurse, one thing you do not want to do after being denied admission to nursing school is to rule out nursing just because you did not get in on the first attempt.

Ask for an Explanation

After you have cooled off, you might consider setting up a time to speak with someone involved with admissions at the institution where you applied. Your goal in this appointment is not to argue that you should have been admitted but to identify areas in your application (e.g., personal statement, letters of reference) that you could strengthen. Assuming you are a qualified applicant, you want to figure how you could make your application showcase your qualifications better.

Get Experience in the Healthcare Field and Reapply

One way you may be able to enhance your application is to take a paid or volunteer position working in the healthcare field. A work or volunteer experience that expands and deepens your perspective on nursing, patient care, and the healthcare system is likely to make you a more attractive nursing school candidate. Moreover, it is possible that you will be able to write a more compelling personal statement based on this experience and you may be able to network with healthcare professionals who will be able to provide you with a recommendation for nursing school.

Take Prerequisites

Assuming that you have not taken some or all of your prerequisite courses, you might consider taking prerequisites courses such as anatomy and physiology, chemistry, microbiology, and nutrition before reapplying to nursing school. As long as you take courses that meet the requirements for nursing school, you will speed your journey through nursing school. In addition, there is an association between high grades in the prerequisite nursing courses and grades in nursing school and first-time pass rate on the NCLEX. Consequently, if you are successful in these courses, you will demonstrate to admission committees for nursing school that you are able to handle the academic rigors of nursing school.

Retake Science Classes with Poor Grades

If you took a prerequisite nursing course such as anatomy and physiology or organic chemistry and received less than a *B*, you might consider retaking the course before reapplying to nursing school. As discussed, there is an association between grades in science courses and grades in nursing school and first-time pass rate on the NCLEX. You might be able to improve your standing among other nursing school applicants by showing higher marks in prerequisite courses.

Sidebar 4-3

Recommendations for Applying to Nursing School

- *Know the deadlines.* Getting into nursing school is tough enough without turning your application in after the deadline. If your application is postmarked after the deadline, you radically reduce your chances of admission.
- *Plan on submitting ahead of the deadline.* There is no reason to wait until the deadline to submit your application. By planning to submit a week or two ahead of the deadline, you give yourself a cushion against the letter of reference that has not arrived, a problem with your computer, or a family emergency.
- *Keep it simple.* Do not make your application difficult for the admissions office at the nursing school by using different variations of your name or devising your own system for completing the application. Read all instructions prior to beginning your application and follow the instructions to the letter. In addition, include your social security number on your application and your application forms because it helps admission offices. It is also required for financial aid awards.
- *Make copies.* Make a copy of your application and all of the forms that you submit. It is a hassle, but if something gets lost it will save you time in the long run.
- *Online applications.* While many institutions are moving to online applications, there may be some components of your application that have to be mailed in. Make sure to get those documents in by the deadline. In addition, print out online application forms before submitting to make sure that they look good on paper.

References

Leners, D., Beardslee, N. Q., & Peters, D. (1996). 21st century nursing and implications for nursing school admissions. *Nursing Outlook, 44,* 137–140.

PricewaterhouseCoopers' Health Research Institute. (2007). What works: Healing the healthcare staffing shortage. Retrieved July 31, 2007, from http://pwchealth.com/cgi-local/hcregister.cgi?link=reg/pubwhatworks.pdf

Sayles, S., Shelton, D., & Powell, H. (2003). Predictors of success in nursing school. *Association of Black Nursing Faculty Journal, 14,* 116–120.

Stelzer, R. (1989). *How to write a winning personal statement for graduate and professional school.* Princeton, NJ: Peterson's Guides.

Tanabe. G., & Tanabe K. (2007). Acing Your College Interview. Retrieved August 6, 2007, from http://www.quintcareers.com/collegeinterview.html

Yin, T., & Burger, C. (2003). Predictors of NCLEX-RN success of associate degree nursing graduates. *Nurse Educator, 28,* 232–236.

APPENDIX 4-A

Sample Admission Essay with Critique

Essay Question:
Indicate a person who has had a significant influence on you and describe that influence.

"We are now in America; anything you want you can get, it's not like in the country. I had to eat worms and crickets in order to survive. I crossed many minefields and war zones to get all seven of you here so that you can have a better life than me."

(Vanna Kim, my mother)

Education is for me what coming to America was for my mother—the ticket to a better life. I grew up in Camden, New Jersey, currently the country's poorest, and one of its most violent, cities. Like most very poor cities, Camden has a failing education system. I was extremely fortunate that my 6th-grade teacher took note of

> **COMMENT:**
> *Good.* The applicant does a great job of capturing the reader's attention and making herself distinct from other applicants with this personal quotation because she lets the reader know that her experiences (or at least those of her mother) are different from most of her peers.

> **COMMENT:**
> *Good.* The first sentence of this paragraph, in conjunction with the initial quotation, give the reader a sense that the theme of this essay will be educational opportunity and her mother's influence as a role model.

> **COMMENT:**
> *Not so good.* The applicant should avoid making claims that might be controversial and/or hard to substantiate.

my academic interest and recommended me to Mullica Hill Friends School, a private institution. Mullica Hill offered me a full scholarship, which I was overjoyed to accept. To attend school at Mullica Hill required a big commitment in time. Each day required four hours of commuting to and from school via public transportation. I began my bus trip at 5:30 a.m. and arrived home each day at 5:30 p.m. The opportunity was well worth all the commuting time. The learning environment at Mullica Hill was quite exciting, and I learned a lot. Mullica Hill also helped me obtain a scholarship for Solebury School, a small boarding school in Pennsylvania. My illiterate mother, who spent her childhood in Cambodia, could have only dreamed of such an opportunity.

My mother's struggles taught me that nothing is impossible. She is my role model; I intend to take full advantage of the opportunities that her efforts have made available to me. My mother's life instills in me a desire to obtain the best possible education and to use that education to contribute to the well-being of others, to "rise with the occasion" as Abraham Lincoln wrote. Over the last few years, I have been contributing to the welfare of those who live in Camden. I have become a leader in the STARR (Sports Teaching Adolescents Responsibility and Resiliency) Program, of which I have been a member since I was in sixth grade. The program is outside of school and is year-round; its purpose is to keep kids away from the streets, drugs, and violence. The program nurtures the development of responsibility and resiliency in children, and their ability to form a meaningful relationship through sports, community services, and academic mentors.

COMMENT:

Good. The applicant keeps the focus of the essay very personal.

COMMENT:

Not so good. The essay could have been organized better. The discussion of Camden and her trips to private school are interesting but do not belong in the introduction.

COMMENT:

Not so good. The role of the applicant's mother as a role model belongs in the introduction.

COMMENT:

Good. The applicant highlights her community service activities and, more importantly, gives concrete examples of what she has done to enhance the welfare of others.

I was once a youth who needed every element of support the program offered; I'm now someone who contributes back to the program. As a youth leader in the program, I model the importance of contributing to the community in our regular service projects such as picking up trash at local schools and parks, planting trees with the New Jersey Tree Foundation, delivering turkey baskets to needy families for Thanksgiving, walking to raise money for lupus research, and sorting food at the South Jersey Food Bank. I know that when younger kids see me working hard in these efforts and listen to me talking about why these actions are important that they are encouraged to think of themselves as active citizens contributing to the welfare of our city.

I need to become much smarter if I'm to make the contributions that are my dream. Consequently, I vow to take every opportunity given to me by xxxx xxxxx College to assist in the building of its community and my character. A great philosopher once said, "You cannot step twice into the same river." I agree. Unlike many other schools, xxxx xxxxx College offers a small faculty-to-student ratio, state-of-the-art facilities, over a hundred clubs, and faculty accessibility. If you admit me to your college, I am certain that these opportunities will offer a unique experience necessary for my personal as well as my academic growth, giving me the chance for the transformation of a lifetime.

COMMENT:

Not so good. The applicant failed to relate her community service activity to the overall theme of the essay—her mother as a role model and educational opportunity.

COMMENT:

Not so good. The applicant could have probably done a better job of condensing this section.

COMMENT:

Not so good. The applicant does not specify what her "dream" or career aspirations are and how this college can assist her in achieving that dream.

COMMENT:

Not so good. Be careful with quotations like this that are not immediately clear to the reader.

COMMENT:

Not so good. The reader knows what the strengths of the college are. What the reader may be interested in understanding is how the applicant's strengths mesh with those of the college and how the applicant might add to the college. For example, the applicant wants to become a nurse so she might have spent some time discussing the nursing program's reputation.

COMMENT:

Not so good. The applicant concluded with a fairly generic and bland concluding sentence (and paragraph). The applicant could have used the conclusion to connect her experiences working with others in community service to her future goals of working with others as a nurse.

Critique:

As you can see from the comments, although there are clear strengths to this essay (e.g., the applicant has an interesting background and experiences, the essay is personal), there are a number of problems. One of the fundamental problems is that the applicant fails to answer the question given in the prompt. The applicant is supposed to write about a role model and the influence that this role model has had upon her. While the applicant clearly indicates that her mother has been a role model, the applicant does not explain how her mother has influenced her educational aspirations and desire to use her education to contribute to the well-being of others. The applicant should have discussed how the mother views education and service to others. The applicant could have also discussed what her mother thought about her decision to pursue a career in nursing.

In addition, the reader has to do too much work to make out the overall theme of this essay. Readers of admission essays have to read several essays in a sitting and, in turn, are most likely to rate most favorably the essays in which the applicant has clearly articulated the theme of the essay. Applicants should assume that the reader of their essay has neither the time nor the patience to figure out the central theme of their essay. The applicant who wrote this essay vacillates between the themes of educational opportunity and her mother as a role model but fails to connect the two. There are a number of interesting points that the applicant mentions; however, I found myself asking, "What is the applicant trying to say here?"

APPENDIX 4-B

Sample Admission Letter with Critique

The reason why I have selected Nursing as a career is because it is a job where you can take pride in your work. Nursing is a career where you can go home every day feeling that you have accomplished something, where, I feel a lot of jobs don't offer that. It has also come to my understanding that it is a secure job and the need for quality nurses has increased over the past few years.

I have chosen the Cochran School of Nursing for several reasons. Throughout my search for a quality school that offers the RN program, the Cochran School of Nursing continuously appeared. I also heard from other students while taking the Anatomy and Physiology I program that "Cochran" was a school to surely be taken into consideration.

COMMENT:

The applicant gets off to a good start by responding immediately to the stated question: Why do you want to become a nurse?

COMMENT:

The writer tries to make three points about why he wanted to become a nurse: job to be proud of, sense of accomplishment with providing care, and job security. Unfortunately, the writing is kind of clunky and, in turn, the reader might get distracted, which is a negative in an admission letter. A more effective introduction might have started like this:

There are couple of reasons that I chose nursing as a career. One reason is that, in contrast to other career choices, nurses make a difference in the lives of people and I want to go home every day feeling that I made a difference. In addition, I like the fact that because of the need for nurses in the health-care system, I will have job security.

I already have a Bachelor's degree in Psychology and I am hoping to use this to my advantage once I become an RN. I also consider myself to be a very determined person. I have been holding two jobs since I have gotten out of college and had to drop the "off the books" job in order to start attending night school. I don't feel that holding an Associate Degree in Nursing will be enough for me; I can surely see myself taking classes to get a Bachelor and maybe even going for a Masters in a certain field. I'm not sure which field it will be, so, I want to take my time once I am a Nurse to see which part of being an RN gives me the greatest amount of satisfaction. I would be very thankful for getting into this program, if not in the Fall semester, then the Spring. Thank you for your time and consideration.

Sincerely Yours,

John Smith

COMMENT:

The letter would have flowed smoother if the applicant used a transitional sentence like, I have a number of strengths that will contribute to my success in nursing school and as a nurse.

COMMENT:

This sentence could be re-worded so that it does not offend nurses who have not gone on for a baccalaureate degree in nursing.

COMMENT:

I don't think this sentence adds much to the letter.

Critique:

Overall, this letter is fairly coherent and the applicant does a good job of providing the reader with a personal account of why he is going into nursing, why he chose this particular school, and what his future plans are.

The applicant did a fair job of personalizing the letter. This is an important point to remember in writing admission letters: your letter is a substitute for a personal interview, so try to include information that the reader will probably not be able to pick up in the admission application. Generate some interest in you as an applicant by adding personal details like "I have been holding two jobs since I have gotten out of college."

In addition, the applicant does a good job of providing specific information about himself (e.g., determined person, working two jobs).

A clear weakness of this letter is that, while the letter is organized and coherent, some of the writing is clunky. For example, the applicant wrote: "I can surely see myself taking classes to get a Bachelor and maybe even going for a Masters in a certain field."

FIVE

The Nursing School Courses

All nursing school graduates must take the same licensing exam; consequently, there is substantial overlap in what nursing school students study. Where diploma, associate, and baccalaureate nursing programs differ is in clinical experience—students in diploma and associate degree programs get more clinical experience than their counterparts in baccalaureate programs—and in emphasis—students in baccalaureate programs receive additional education in liberal arts, leadership and management, and community nursing. In this section I discuss the clinical theory courses, the science courses, and the nonscience courses that you may take in nursing school.

Clinical Theory Courses

Most of the clinical theory courses are half a semester long, and they are paired with your clinical experience. The purpose of the clinical theory courses is to provide you with the theoretical and scientific basis for making clinical decisions that pertain to the population for whom you are providing care. A substantial portion of the course is spent discussing the major health problems that affect the various populations and the interventions to restore health. In addition, you will also learn evidence-based strategies to promote and maintain the health of this population. The names of the clinical theory courses vary by institution, but the basic courses are briefly discussed below.

- Nursing fundamentals—In this course you are introduced to the fundamental nursing concepts, skills, and techniques. A primary aim of this course is to assist you in developing your critical thinking abilities and your ability to utilize the nursing process. In addition, you will learn to apply fundamental nursing skills, including therapeutic communication, assessing vital signs, calculation of drug doses, and medication administration via oral, topical, subcutaneous, and intramuscular routes.
- Health assessment—During this semester-long course you will learn and practice the skills you will need to perform a check for vital signs (blood pressure, pulse, temperature, and respirations), a mental status check, and a thorough head-to-toe assessment of all the major systems. You will learn to use a stethoscope (most schools require you to purchase your own nurse pack containing all the health assessment tools you will need for the semester such as stethoscope, sphygmomanometer, otoscope, reflex hammer, and penlight). Most programs are evenly divided between two hours of lecture and two hours of hands-on instruction in the lab practicing the skills you have been taught on a partner.
- Nursing care of children—In this course you will learn about the common subacute, acute, and chronic health problems of children and the role of nurses as part of a multidisciplinary team in managing these problems. Moreover, you will develop an understanding of normal patterns of growth and development from infancy through adolescence.
- Nursing care of adults—As you might guess from the title, the focus of this course is on adults and you will learn about providing caring that promotes, maintains, and restores health in adults.
- Nursing care of the child-bearing family—In this course you learn all about childbirth—from conception through delivery.
- Nursing care of the aged—Aging brings about a number of physiological changes that influence health, and in this course you will learn about those changes.

- Nursing care of individuals with mental health problems—In this course you learn about the range of mental health diagnoses and the different treatments for individuals experiencing mental health problems.
- Community health—Students taking the baccalaureate route will also take a community health course. The goal of this course is to provide you with an understanding of the various roles nurses serve in promoting, maintaining, and restoring health in the community. These roles include home care, hospice nursing, and school nursing.
- Nursing leadership—As noted above, this type of course is specific to baccalaureate programs and provides students with an overview of contemporary leadership and management theories. The emphasis is on understanding the key skills employed by successful nurse leaders/managers, such as critical thinking, effective communication, conflict resolution, team building, and leading change.

Sidebar 5-1

Courses in Nursing Require More Than Courses in Other Majors

I teach in an associate degree program at a community college, and most of our students tend to be second-career students or adults who have to work while they attend school because they are paying their own tuition. Students in our program take courses part-time. We have found that during the prerequisite phase of the nursing program many of our students are able to complete the prerequisite classes (e.g., English, sociology) without much trouble. In contrast, when these students get to the nursing courses, the work load is much different. In their nursing courses they have at least 4 hours of lecture every week that requires them to do the reading in advance, and there is a laboratory requirement where students have to perform nursing-related skills. As they progress through the curriculum and begin the clinical nursing courses, the time demands become even greater. Not only are students performing 16 hours of clinical study every week, but they must allot time to prepare for the clinical work, and travel back and forth to the clinical site. We have found that the quicker students realize that nursing courses are more demanding than courses in other majors and the importance of prioritizing their nursing studies, the better they do as nursing students.

Carol Carofiglio, PhD, RN
Nursing Faculty
Helene Fuld School of Nursing In Camden County

Science Courses

Microbiology

In this course you will study microbes, which are single cell and multi-cell organisms that are everywhere but cannot be seen without microscopes or other magnification devices. In addition to learning about the basic types of microbes (prokaryotic and eukaryotic), you will learn about the beneficial and detrimental effects these microbes can have on the body and how we attempt to control these various microbes. Part of your learning about microbiology occurs through spending time in the lab studying microorganisms. During this time you will grow, examine, and characterize some basic microbes.

Inorganic Chemistry

Depending on the program, this course may be combined with organic chemistry to form a one-semester course or it may be offered as a one-semester course of its own. Either way you will learn the basic concepts of chemistry, with special reference to inorganic compounds, including chemical equations, the periodic table, and chemical bonding. In this one-semester course you will be required to perform mathematic calculations involving exponential numbers and scientific notation and to solve word problems involving percent ratios and proportions. In the laboratory component of the course, you will put on goggles and lab coat as you mix chemicals and fire up the Bunsen burner. There are a number of different inorganic chemistry courses offered at colleges and universities, and to save yourself time make sure that whatever inorganic chemistry you take meets the requirements for the nursing program you are considering. This is one of those courses that can cause problems for students when they try to transfer because it may deal with inorganic chemistry but not include the lab that is required for nursing, or it may be a course that is designed for science majors, who have a better understanding of the subject matter than do nursing majors.

Sidebar 5-2

Recommendation for Students Who Are Unsure About Science

If you did not take high school chemistry or biology, it's been many years since your high school chemistry or biology courses, or you did not do well in high school chemistry or biology, consider taking a noncredit course in college usually called "developmental chemistry" or "developmental biology." The purpose of these types of courses is to prepare you for the college-level chemistry or college-level biology courses. These additional courses may lengthen the time it takes for you to graduate; however, you will get more out of the required science course, when you take it. At the very least, in the weeks before you begin taking a science course, "brush up" on scientific terms and concepts by reviewing a science book or looking at some of the many resources available on the internet.

Jeanne Ruggiero, PhD, RN, APN-C
Assistant Professor, College of Nursing
Seton Hall University

Organic Chemistry

As discussed, depending on the program, this course may be a one-semester course or combined with inorganic chemistry. The aim of this course is to provide you with the foundation in biochemistry and molecular genetics you will need as a nurse. The focus of organic chemistry is on normal cell metabolism and the uses of organic and biological compounds in health-related situations. Many students have difficulty with this course because success requires that one stay on top of the material. By staying on top of the material, I mean reviewing the concepts discussed in class, memorizing, and working practice problems. The nice part of organic chemistry is that most professors relate it to nursing by discussing some of the biologic and organic compounds involved in health-related situations. As with inorganic chemistry, most nursing schools require that your organic chemistry has a lab component.

Anatomy and Physiology

Most nursing schools require two semesters of anatomy and physiology (A&P) for their students along with a weekly lab. In A&P courses you learn the structure (anatomy) of the body's organs, skeleton, muscles, nerves, and how all of the systems in the body function together (physiology) to allow us to breathe, digest food, think, and procreate. Although this course can be challenging, most students find it interesting because it gives one a whole new appreciation for the human body.

Nutrition

Depending on the program, this course may be integrated throughout the curriculum (e.g., content offered in other courses such as *Nursing Care of Children*) or offered as a one-semester course on its own. As you might expect in a course titled nutrition, the focus is on the basics of human nutrition. Talking about food is not a bad way to spend a semester, and I do not recall ever hearing someone say, "I hated nutrition."

You pick up all sorts of interesting information (e.g., there are 3,500 calories per pound of body fat), and you learn to read food labels critically. Moreover, you learn how nutritional needs change through the life cycle and the relationship between nutrition and health.

Pathophysiology

In addition to the science courses discussed above, some schools—typically baccalaureate programs—require pathophysiology. If you take this course, you will study functional changes associated with or resulting from disease or injury. It would be impossible to study all diseases, so most of these courses focus on the most common diseases for each body system, such as hypertension for the heart, diabetes for the endocrine system, and asthma for the lungs.

Pharmacology

This is another one of those courses which, depending on the program, may be integrated throughout the curriculum or offered as a one-semester course. In this course you learn about the different categories of medications such as antibiotics, drugs for hypertension, and drugs to manage pain. You will not be able to open up your own pharmacy after completing pharmacology; however, you will be very familiar with the more commonly used drugs and have a basic understanding of how the drugs work, their important side effects, and contraindications.

Other Courses

There are also some other courses that you may be required to take depending on the school that you attend and the path that you take to becoming a registered nurse.

Research Methods

This semester-long course is specific to baccalaureate programs. Your time is spent learning the research process, learning to critique articles from research journals, discussing the ethical aspects of research, and beginning to learn the difference between types of research design. This is one of the courses that I teach, and I have found that the greatest challenge of this course for students is learning the terms that are used in research, such as *validity*, *reliability*, and *qualitative design*. The students who do well are those who commit themselves to learning the terminology of research.

Statistics
This course is also specific to baccalaureate programs and usually includes the same content whether you take it at Harvard or your local community college. In this course you learn about descriptive statistics (e.g., mean, median, and mode), probability, and inferential statistics, which are used to make generalizations from a sample to a population. For most students statistics courses are challenging because, while these courses are similar to math courses, the basic concepts are not intuitive for most people.

Introduction to Psychology
The name of the course varies by institution, but the content usually includes a review of the major emotional, cognitive, and social developments that occur from birth to death (womb to the tomb). The theories of individuals such as Freud, Erickson, and Piaget are used to guide your thinking about human development. Depending on the course, content on physical development may also be included.

English Composition I & II
These two courses focus on preparing you to write the traditional academic essays (e.g., research papers) that you will be assigned as a nursing student. They are one-semester courses and are required in most nursing programs.

Introduction to Sociology
Depending on your nursing program, this course may not be required. The primary purpose of this course is to provide you with some of the basic concepts of sociology and an understanding of how sociological research is conducted.

Ethics/Philosophy
This course is not required in all nursing programs and the content varies by nursing program. In most programs this course provides students with an introduction to ethical theory and practice, with a focus on its application to the nursing profession.

SIX

You and Your Professor

For a variety of reasons you and your professor are probably not going to become best friends, drinking buddies, or travel cross country together for spring break; however, when you graduate from nursing school and become a registered nurse, you and your nursing school professors will be colleagues in the profession of nursing. Consequently, it makes sense to make an effort to get along with your professors in nursing school. Moreover, establishing an amicable relationship with your professors is important because your professor may be able to provide support as you progress through nursing school and begin your career. A professor with whom you have an amicable relationship will be more likely to take into consideration an emergency situation (e.g., illness, death in the family) that would make it difficult for you to take an exam. That professor is much more likely to supply a letter of reference that you will need for graduate school.

Classroom Etiquette

One way to develop a poor relationship with your professor is to disrupt the classroom environment with your actions or your words. Consequently, it is in

Sidebar 6-1

Don't Be Anonymous

Students should make an effort to get to know the faculty who teach their courses. Faculty are interested in getting to know students, but many of the classes in nursing schools have a great number of students and unless students make the effort it is hard to connect faces with names. Taking the time to introduce yourself to the instructors in your course has at least two benefits: First, it is easier to get a letter of reference for graduate school or a job if the professor knows who you are, and secondly, if you are struggling with a class or have a personal emergency, it is easier to approach your instructor if you have taken the time earlier in the semester to establish a relationship with that faculty member.

Cynthia Ayres, PhD, RN
Assistant Professor, College of Nursing
Rutgers, The State University of New Jersey

your best interest and the best interest of your fellow students to do your best to avoid creating friction in the classroom. How does one create friction in the classroom environment? The following sections discuss some ways.

Arriving Late to Class

It is unlikely that you want to be disruptive. In fact, you may not even be aware that by showing up to class late you are being disruptive. However, you should know that it is easy to lose one's train of thought when giving a lecture, and it is just as easy to lose the audience's attention. Both of these outcomes are likely to occur when a student enters the class late. To get a sense of what type of disruption lateness causes in a class, especially a small class, take notice of your professor's reaction and the reaction of other students when other students arrive late to class. The instructor and students lose focus as they take notice of the new arrival.

Real-World Snapshot 6-1

Advice for Students Having Difficulty

Do not wait until the end of the semester to approach the professor of a class in which you are having trouble. In most cases it is too late by the end of the semester for the professor to be of any assistance.

Jeanne Ruggiero, PhD, RN, APN-C
Assistant Professor, College of Nursing
Seton Hall University

Distracting Classroom Behaviors

As mentioned, it is easy to get distracted during a lecture—both for the lecturer and the audience—and, while instant messaging on one's cell phone, reading the newspaper, eating, stretching, carrying on a quiet conversation, and passing notes may seem like activities that would not be noticed by your professor, they are noticed. Despite the fact that your professor may be standing in the front of the room barricaded behind a lectern armed with an LCD projector and PowerPoint slides, it is hard *not* to notice what is happening in the room. An instructor knows if he or she has the attention of the class. Distracting actions such as those mentioned above are likely to annoy your professor, your fellow students, and spoil the classroom environment.

Discourteous or Inflammatory Questions or Remarks

In addition to disrupting the classroom environment through behaviors, one can also upset the classroom environment and, in turn, the learning process, through what one says. In class (and out of class), it is important to choose one's words carefully and to make sure that what you say is not disrespectful of your fellow students or your professor. Of course, comments that are disrespectful of other students or your professor or reflect intolerance have no place in the classroom and may result in disciplinary action. However, even when the comments one makes do not violate the standards of classroom behavior, it is worth thinking about how to communicate in class. For example, consider a situation in which your professor made a point during a lecture that you do not agree with or that conflicts with your experiences, such as "Children should not sleep in the same bed as their parents." Raising your hand and saying something like, "Everybody knows that co-sleeping is healthy," or "I don't see how you can say something like that," may be interpreted as aggressive or adversarial and may cause a negative or defensive response from

Sidebar 6-2

Inappropriate Classroom Behaviors

- Using laptops and other Web-enabled digital devices to check e-mail and browse the Web (e.g., YouTube). Some faculty will notice your subsequent lack of attention to the class and assume that you are engaging in these behaviors.
- Reading or sending text messages during class
- Cell phones that are not set to vibrate during class
- Talking to other students during a lecture portion of class
- Reading the newspaper or other reading material during class

Jeanne Ruggiero, PhD, RN, APN-C
Assistant Professor,
College of Nursing
Seton Hall University

your instructor. On the other hand, saying something framed more positively, such as, "Would you mind expanding on your last point regarding co-sleeping?" or "Could you clarify that point?" is more likely to stimulate a productive discussion and less likely to cause disruption.

Communicating with Your Professor

In addition to developing skills that will enhance communication between you and your professor in the classroom, there are also ways to enhance communication between you and your professor outside of the classroom. You may be thinking, "Why would I ever want to speak with my professor outside of the classroom?" As discussed, you and your professor are probably not going to be best buddies, but you are a nursing colleague in training and your professor can give you insight into the profession. In addition, your professor can provide guidance and advisement regarding difficult course concepts and assignments that he or she is teaching. As discussed, most nursing school professors are busy with the other aspects of their job, such as scholarly research or clinical practice; however, most nursing faculty went into education because they enjoy working with students, and they look forward to talking with students. Take advantage of the opportunity to talk with your nursing school professor outside of the classroom. In most nursing schools your professor will post office hours. If the scheduled times do not fit with your schedule you should contact your professor about scheduling an alternative time.

Sidebar 6-3

How to Handle Personal Problems or Family Crises That May Arise During Nursing School

If you have problems or life issues, speak with your instructor as early as possible. Do not hold back and cut classes, and don't be mysterious. When faculty do not see students in class and they do not know otherwise, they assume the students are cutting class because they do not care. But when a student tells me that they are having family issues or some problem going on outside of school, I can give them an extension on a paper or let them delay taking an exam. I want students to pass; I do not want to fail students, but I can only help them if they let me know what is going on.

Jeanne Ruggiero, PhD, RN, APN-C
Assistant Professor, College of Nursing
Seton Hall University

Office Hours

Although most professors enjoy meeting with their students, you should come to the office hours prepared to discuss your specific issues or concerns. There is nothing wrong with preparing a short list of questions or issues that you have. In fact, your meeting might be more productive if you share the issues that you want to discuss during your meeting ahead of the meeting. Besides being prepared, you should be on time for your meeting (being a little early isn't bad either), and make sure that you thank your instructor for his or her time. What shouldn't you do? You shouldn't miss a scheduled meeting without informing your professor. If you know that you cannot make it to the meeting, let your professor know as far in advance as possible.

If your purpose for meeting with your professor is to discuss a grade, give yourself a "cooling off" period after receiving the grade before scheduling a meeting. You shouldn't discuss the grade you received on a test or assignment when you are angry or upset. The cooling off period will allow you to get some emotional distance before meeting with your professor. You will be better able to focus on the reason that you think your grade was assigned unfairly rather than on the grade. Most professors do not enjoy haggling over grades, but they do care that you learn, and they do care about fairness.

In an ideal world, you and your professor would be able to have a face-to-face conversation whenever the need arose. Unfortunately for most nursing students and faculty, work schedules, class schedules, and geographical distance

Sidebar 6-4

Keep Your Professor in the Loop

This past semester I had one student who did not submit her paper by the deadline. When I realized that the student had not submitted her paper I became concerned, and I contacted the student to get an explanation. The student responded that she had a "lot going on with work," and she wasn't able to complete the assignment. I wish this student had contacted me when she realized she was going to have difficulty in meeting the deadline. I may have been able to consider an extension. However, because the paper was not submitted on time, to be fair to the students in the class who met the deadline, I had to deduct points off the paper for each day it was late, and the student ended up getting a poor grade. This story underscores the importance of keeping professors in the loop and establishing a relationship with the professor. We understand that sometimes personal problems or emergencies arise, and we are willing to give extensions if we know of a problem in advance.

Cynthia Ayres, PhD, RN
Assistant Professor,
College of Nursing Rutgers,
The State University of New Jersey

Sidebar 6-5

Don't Harass Professors About Grades

Most of your professors in nursing school are teaching more than one course, and while we understand that you want to know your grades in the course or on a particular assignment, we are doing our best to grade assignments as quickly and efficiently as possible. Inquiries regarding grades via phone calls, e-mails, or office visits do nothing to expedite the grading and only add to your professor's stress level.

Cynthia Ayres, PhD, RN
Assistant Professor, College of Nursing
Rutgers, The State University of New Jersey

Sidebar 6-6

Your Nursing School Handbook

Nursing school student handbooks all have policies and procedures that you will need to know about your school. Read it carefully, keep it handy, and refer to it often. Course syllabi are also extremely important. Read them carefully, and refer to them often to avoid missing course requirements that may lead to a low or failing grade. Don't wait until the week before the semester ends. It is often too late to fix a problem.

Jeanne Ruggiero, PhD, RN, APN-C
Assistant Professor, College of Nursing
Seton Hall University

---

make it difficult to schedule face-to-face meetings. Consequently, when you need to communicate with your professor outside of class, you may have to rely on e-mail or voice mail. Virtually all nursing school faculty have access to institutional e-mail and voice mail accounts, and most encourage their students to communicate with them using these technologies. In the sections that follow are tips on how to improve communication with your faculty when using e-mail and voice mail.

Real-World Snapshot 6-2

If You Have a Concern About How
a Grade Was Assigned

When you contact your professor, keep the following in mind: Do not discuss how your grade was assigned during class; do it privately after class with him or her. Do not criticize the professor's grade distribution, grading system, and so on. If you plan to contact your professor via e-mail, I recommend that you write a draft of your e-mail and save it to review before you send it. It is appropriate for you to be angry and upset with a lower grade than you expected, but do not send an e-mail in this state. Once you send an angry, accusatory e-mail it cannot be retrieved.

Review your student handbook to see if your concern is addressed in the handbook.

Schedule a time to meet with the faculty member who assigned your grade. Do not let this discussion become an argument. Ask for the faculty member's rationale or evidence for assigning the grade under dispute. Many faculty are not going to be accessible during the holiday break, so don't expect a response to an e-mail you sent on Christmas Eve. You may not hear back until after New Year's Day or later. This is why it is so important to be on top of your performance in the course throughout the semester. If you wait until the end of the semester and then ask your professor for special treatment (e.g., a paper to boost your grade from failing to passing), your request is unlikely to be honored.

If after meeting with the faculty member who assigned your grade, you believe that an error was made or your grade was assigned unfairly, consult your student handbook to determine the process for resolving grade disputes. Follow this process, which may include filing a written complaint with the department chair. Follow the chain of command in order to present a positive and professional image of yourself. Do not go above your professor's "head" unless you have communicated with him or her first.

Although it is appropriate for you to be assertive and on top of your grades, and to be disappointed if you did not do well in a course, it is not appropriate to argue with your professor, challenge his or her authority, go above his or her head (that person will refer you back), or to blame him or her for your difficulties and performance in the course. You may have this professor in another course or need a letter of recommendation in the future. You want him or her to remember you in a positive light.

Jeanne Ruggiero, PhD, RN, APN-C
*Assistant Professor, College of Nursing
Seton Hall University*

E-Mail Etiquette

It is likely that most readers of this book are very comfortable using e-mail and voice mail; however, as Jonathan Glater reported in his *New York Times* article, "To: Professor@University.edu Subject: Why it's all about me" (Glater, 2006), many students do not recognize that what they say in their voice mails or write in their e-mails may adversely affect their relationship with their professor. Moreover, as Glater points out, "The barrage of e-mail has brought new tension" into the work lives of professors. I am sure that stressing out their professors is not the goal of most students, certainly not nursing students. A discussion on e-mail and voice mail etiquette is provided below.

The following do's and don'ts on e-mail etiquette are adapted from suggestions provided at the Web site *Emailreplies.com* (Emailreplies.com, n.d.). I have revised these suggestion based on e-mails I have received as a professor in nursing school. We will begin by looking at two sample e-mails that I received from students over the past few years that do not make a good impression. All identifying information has been removed from the e-mails. I included these e-mails to give concrete examples of why it is important to adhere to some basic rules when e-mailing your professors and others:

Subject: Nursing Research
From: janedoe@verizon.com
To: robert.atkins@rutgers.edu

HI PROF ATKINS, IN UNIT x THREADED DISCUSSION, I WROTE ON THE XXXXXX CASE, I HOPE THAT,S OKAY WITH YOU. ALSO,PLS USE MY "SCHOOL" E-MAIL ACCOUNT OR JANEDOE@YAHOO.COM. THE E-MAILS SENT TO VERIZON ARE NOT BEEN RECIEVED.

THANKS.
JANE DOE

Subject: Nursing Research
From: John Doe
To: Robert.atkins@rutgers.edu

doc,
hey i was wondering if i could do my research paper on yawning and why it is contagious

The Do's for E-Mail

Do Use Proper Spelling, Grammar, and Punctuation

It may seem like a petty issue to emphasize, but your professor probably receives more e-mail each day than he or she would like to receive. If your professor is anything like me, he or she wants to get through them as quickly and efficiently as possible. Receiving e-mails like the ones above that have errors in spelling, punctuation, and grammar are not likely to brighten his or her day or make a great impression. These types of e-mails are difficult to read quickly and sometimes the message gets lost. Your friends and family that receive sloppy and informal e-mails do not care, but it is in your best interest to take the extra time necessary to read your e-mail over and correct errors in spelling, grammar, and punctuation.

Do Be Concise and to the Point

As discussed above, your professor is trying to get through e-mail as quickly and efficiently as possible, and reading an e-mail is not like reading printed communication. Keep your sentences short (maximum 15–20 words), and make it clear in your e-mail why you are writing: What do you want? Are you asking for an extension on a paper? Clarification of a point made in class? A letter of reference? If you have a number of questions that require

---

Sidebar 6-7

Recommendations for Addressing Your Faculty in Nursing School

If a faculty member in your nursing program has earned a doctorate, such as a Doctor of Philosophy (PhD), Doctor of Education (EdD), or Doctor of Nursing Science (DNS), address that individual using the title of doctor (e.g., Dr. Smith). When addressing faculty members in your nursing program who have not earned a doctorate, or in situations in which you are unsure of the educational background of a faculty member, address the individual as Professor (e.g., Professor Smith). Faculty who have earned doctorates usually do not mind being addressed as Professor either. In some institutions, faculty who are at the instructor level are referred to as "Mr." or "Mrs./Ms./Miss." In some clinical settings the faculty will allow you to address them by first name, but do not assume that it is alright to do so— everyone is different. These suggestions are applicable to both verbal and written communication. Start your e-mail with "Dear Prof. X" or simply, "Prof. X." Avoid starting the e-mail with "hey," or without the professor's title and last name. While e-mail is a universally acceptable form of communication, e-mails to professors should not be composed the same way as e-mails to friends and family. The important thing to remember is to be respectful. Also, there is nothing wrong with asking the faculty member how he or she would like to be addressed.

Jeanne Ruggiero, PhD, RN, APN-C
Assistant Professor, College of Nursing
Seton Hall University

substantial explanation, consider using your e-mail to set up a time to discuss your questions in person or over the phone.

For example, read the text of this less than succinct e-mail:

Subject: Recommendation
From: jdoe@verizon.com
To: robert.atkins@rutgers.edu

Hi Dr. Atkins,

How are you? Hope all is well. I am emailing you because both XXXX and I really miss you as our Research teacher and I need a favor ;) I am applying for a teaching position at XXXXX XXXXXX XXXXXXX. Since I only have my BSN, I can only teach in the lab as a lab instructor, but I have put in an application for clinical instructor once I finish my Masters. I need a letter of recommendation from you. 'Cause you're just so awesome! You could send it to my home address and I will hand deliver it to the school with my two other letters of recommendation. My address is as follows:

[DELETED]

Thanks so much. I also had another question. I finish all my general Masters courses at the end of this year, and I start clinical next spring. Do you think Dean XXXXXX would give me like a certificate saying that I am "Masters prepared" since all my general MSN courses would be complete and I will take post-Graduate classes after that towards my NP? Because I know Rutgers doesn't have just a general MSN program—only either CLincal specialist or NP. So if I ask Dean XXXXXX for such a certificate saying that I am essentially Masters prepared minus the clinical component of the NP, do you think that's possible? Just wondering...

Sorry if inundated you with a long email.. I'm sure you are swamped with end of the semester stuff to do too. I would really appreciate the letter of recommendation—as soon as you can...

Again, thank you so much.

Sincerely,
Jdoe

Of course, I read this entire e-mail because my former student said I was "awesome," and I cannot pass up that kind of feedback; however, this e-mail was rather lengthy, and the student would have probably been better off using the e-mail to schedule a time for us to talk in person or over the phone.

Do Give Your Text Room to Breathe

Reading from the computer screen is more difficult than reading from a book or sheet of paper; thus, it is important that you compose your e-mail with short paragraphs and blank lines between each paragraph. For example, the e-mail included above was too long, but if the student had provided some more line spacing it would have been easier for me to deduce exactly what this student wanted.

Do Use a Meaningful Subject Line

As discussed, your professor has to sort through a great deal of e-mail. You can make this task of sorting simpler by including a subject line that suggests who you are and what you want.

Below is an e-mail that is concise, well-spaced, and has a meaningful subject line.

> Subject: Student Advisement Fall 2005
> From: Jane Doe
> To: Robert.atkins@rutgers.edu
>
> Hi Prof Atkins,
> I'd like to schedule a quick meeting with you.
>
> The best for me would be March 25th 3:30 at Bartlett; however, I do have a class at Richardson scheduled from 1–3:40. Let me know what you think.
>
> Thanks,
> Jane Doe

Do Leave the Original Message in the E-Mail in Your Replies

When you leave the original message in your e-mail, you save your professor's time because he or she does not have to recall what was said in the original e-mail or search for the original e-mail to determine what was said.

Do Use Your Student E-mail Account to Send E-mail

When corresponding with faculty, use your student e-mail account instead of a home e-mail account. Your student e-mail account is less likely to be confused as spam or junk mail by your professor. Furthermore, student e-mail accounts are less likely to have screen names—hotmama1290@yahoo.com or boogerboy92@gmail.com—that befuddle faculty who have to determine the sender of the e-mail. If you cannot use your student e-mail account for some reason, let your professor know as soon as possible and consider getting a home account or a free Gmail account with a screen name that incorporates your last name (e.g., ratkins@gmail.com). Overall, however, the best e-mail is your student account because it is the most reliable.

Do Check Your E-mail Every Day
Make sure you check your e-mail every day, even if you tend to use an alternative way of communicating. Some faculty communicate almost entirely by e-mail, and you may miss an important bit of information if you do not take the time to check your account.

The Don'ts for E-Mail

Do Not Forward Chain Letters
You may really like your professor and may feel that you are doing some form of community service by forwarding chain letters with dire warnings of malicious viruses, monetary giveaways from Bill Gates, and urban myths involving kidney harvests; however, these are all hoaxes. Do not forward these chain letters to your professor, your friends, or your family. You are wasting their time, your time, and clogging up the Internet. If you are in doubt about the truth of any of the claims that you receive via e-mail, visit Hoaxbusters.com (http://hoaxbusters.ciac.org/). The administrators of this site do a terrific job of staying abreast of the latest hoaxes circulating on the Internet.

Do Not Forward Religious/Political/Sexual E-mails
While you may have the best of intentions, do not forward e-mail or send e-mail to your professors that contains religious themes (e.g., prayers, angels) or is sexual (e.g., jokes) or political in nature (e.g., petitions to support a politician or political cause). One can never be sure how others will react to this type of e-mail and you run the risk of offending the recipient.

Do Not Use Abbreviations, Emoticons, or ALL CAPITAL LETTERS
Your professor might not be as hip as your friends, so avoid abbreviations and emoticons that might be confusing such as: IMHO (in my humble opinion), LOL (laughing out loud), and MORF (male or female). In addition, use UPPERCASE TEXT only when you want to emphasize a point. Uppercase letters in e-mails are analogous to shouting, and you probably do not want to shout at your professor.

Do Not E-Mail Your Professor to Report That You Are Going to Miss Class or Be Late to Class

Unless your professor has specifically requested that you inform him or her when you are going to miss class or be late, sending an e-mail that explains why you are going to be late or absent only wastes your professor's time. However, it is important to pay close attention to the attendance policies in the nursing program handbook and the syllabus for the course. If class attendance is part of the grade, your professor should have already given you criteria for receiving an excused absence, and you should contact your professor to discuss receiving an excused absence. Of course, if you were scheduled to present something in class and your absence is likely to be disruptive, contact your professor as soon as you know that you will be late.

Do Not E-Mail Your Professor Asking for Class Notes

If you do miss class or you are late and you missed some of the content that was provided, do not ask your professor for a copy of his or her lecture notes. This is not an e-mail that most professors want to receive. Ask one of your peers in the class for a copy of his or her notes.

Do Not E-Mail a Copy of Your Assignment for Your Professor to Provide Feedback

Unless your professor has informed you that you have the option of submitting your assignments early for feedback prior to grading, do not ask your professor to do this for you. Providing feedback on assignments is a time-consuming process, and it is unrealistic to expect that your professor is able to commit to doing this for every student in the course.

Do Not Expect to Receive an Immediate Reply to Your E-Mail

Nursing school faculty will vary in how quickly they respond to you: some will get right back to you; others may take some time. If it is a busy clinical day or your professor is making the final touches on a funding proposal, he or she may be delayed in responding to your e-mail. Sometimes e-mails just get missed, so you may have to follow up. Give your professor at least 24 hours during the working week (even professors deserve some downtime on the weekends) to respond before following up with another e-mail or a phone call. Of course, you improve the likelihood of your professor getting back to you quickly if you make it clear in your e-mail exactly what you want. If you follow the suggestions that have been discussed in this section, you will increase that likelihood.

Voice Mail

The suggestions for voice mail are much briefer than those provided for e-mail. Moreover, some of the tips for e-mail apply to voice mail as well. As with e-mail, it is important to keep in mind that what you say in your voice mail contributes to the impression your professor has of you. Think of what you are going to say before you leave a message. In fact, there is nothing wrong with hanging up the phone and calling back or deleting your message and rerecording if your message does not reflect exactly what you want to say (unfortunately, not all voice mail systems have this feature, so it is best to plan out your message and choose your words carefully). Moreover, remember that your professor, like most business professionals, probably does not love sorting through voice mails. Each voice mail is likely one more item that he is adding to his to-do list. Below are some Do's for voice mail that will help you make a good impression and improve communication between you and your professors.

The Do's for Voice Mail

Do Speak Clearly and Slowly
Factors such as background noise and the quality of the phone connection influence the ease with which your voice mail message is understood. You may not have a great deal of control of the background noise (however, do all you can to limit it) or the quality of the phone equipment, but you can speak clearly and slowly when leaving your message and repeat your number more than once.

Do Leave Your Name and Phone Number
It may be hard to believe, but some students neglect to leave their name (if it is a long name, spell it out) and phone number with their voice mail. Even if your professor recognizes your voice—and that is a big if—he or she will probably not think highly of you if she has to track down your phone number. In some cases your faculty member may not be able to track down your phone number, so take the time at the beginning of the semester to make sure that you give up-to-date contact information to faculty.

Do Be Concise and to the Point
As with e-mail messages, keep your voice mail messages brief. Your friends and family may really enjoy the sound of your voice and may find long rambling voice mails amusing and sweet. It is safe to say that your professor does not. State what you need in the voice mail, and get off the phone. Moreover, do not attempt to pack multiple requests into your voice mail message: one voice mail entitles you to one request.

Do Leave the Date and Time You Called in the Message

Most voice mail systems have time and date stamping of some sort; however, not all have this feature. Thus, it is helpful if you leave a reminder by stating the time and date that you called.

Below are two sample voice mail messages that illustrate how to leave a voice mail and how *not* to leave a voice mail. I have not saved any actual voice mail messages left by students; however, the second voice mail comes close to messages I have received from students.

How to leave a voice mail message:

> Hi, Professor Nightingale, this is Joe Bagofdonuts, a student in your pediatric theory course. It is Monday, April 23rd, at 10:30 a.m., and I am calling because I would like to meet to discuss some questions I have about the evidence-based practice paper assignment that is due next month. You can send me an e-mail or call me back at 856-555-5555 and let me know your next available office hours. Again, this is Joe Bagofdonuts, and my number is 856-555-5555. I look forward to hearing from you. ■

How *not* to leave a voice mail message:

> Hello, hello, Professor Nightingale. This is Joe, and I am leaving you a message because I want to talk to you about the assignment that is due. I was looking at the guidelines last night (dog barking in the background). . . Boffo stop barking. . . my dog is barking because there is someone at my door; I think it is the mailman. The funny thing is the mailman is actually a woman, and she loves animals, but my dog still barks at her. Anyway, like I was saying, I started looking at the guidelines because I hate waiting to the last minute to start working on my assignments— I used to do that in high school, and it drove my parents crazy—and I don't understand if I need to use a clinical issue from my experience or whether I can choose a clinical issue that I think is interesting. I am also not sure whether you want us to use full-out APA and include an abstract in this paper. Most professors don't make us include an abstract, but I don't want to lose points. So if you can call me back, that would be great. My number is 856-555-5555. ■

Obviously, if you were a faculty member you would not want to receive the second voice mail. Even if Joe of the second message spoke clearly, he does not adequately identify himself, he wanders, and he does not leave his number until the end of the voice mail. Moreover, in contrast to the first voice mail, the second voice mail message does not clearly state what the caller wants. Consequently, the faculty member who receives this message will be forced to call back to sort it all out. To avoid creating a game of phone tag, let your professor know what you want so that he or she can give you a response via voice mail if you are not there to answer.

Sidebar 6-8

That Difficult Professor Could Become Your Patient

I clearly remember the shock of finding out that the nursing professor who had made me feel so anxious and unsure as a nursing student was going to be one of my patients. I passed her class, and I never clashed with her, but I, along with many of my peers, felt she was cold, distant, and unapproachable in and out of the classroom while we were students. She was a much better person as a patient than she had been as a professor. As a patient she was warm, funny, and eager to chat about all the things that were going on in her life. In addition, this woman who was so emotionally distant from me and my peers during nursing school wanted to know all about what I had done since I had graduated from nursing school in terms of career and personal life. By the time she was discharged we had formed a nice bond, and I had a hard time believing that this was the same person who had caused me so much torment during my days in nursing school.

Joy Atkins, MA, RN
Adjunct Instructor, Department of Nursing
Rutgers, The State University of New Jersey

Real-World Snapshot 6-3

Nursing Professor Advice

There's a saying out there, "Failure to plan is a plan for failure." Although this saying sounds simple, when it comes to getting the most out of nursing school, this saying is too true. Making a plan is one of the most important things you can do to not only get through nursing school but to lay the foundation for your future endeavors. When you think of being a nursing student, thoughts of long lectures, endless chapter readings, hard tests, and clinical come to mind, I'm sure. Nursing students are so focused on the short-term gratifications, such as getting good grades and getting through clinical, that they do not appreciate other opportunities nursing school has to offer. I don't mean to minimize getting good grades and getting through clinical, as they are extremely important—both a necessity and requirement to being a good nurse and getting through nursing school. However, there are other things that you can get out of nursing school that can help you in the long run—far beyond nursing school. Making a plan for your future is key to a successful nursing career—and it should begin in school.

Your plan should include developing relationships with faculty. These relationships are invaluable. With so many students in your class (times however many other classes your professor is teaching), it is sometimes difficult to remember individual students on a level where a personal or professional reference can be provided for them. This is particularly true when you apply for a nursing position after graduation or apply for graduate school. If a faculty member knows you on a personal level, he or she is better able to discuss your strengths and assets in a letter of recommendation—much more preferable than a general letter of reference for someone they don't remember very well, except for their course grade. In addition, faculty cannot only provide you with recommendations to get into graduate school, but who knows—they may teach you in graduate school as well. I have taught a number of students in the undergraduate program who I have also taught years later in graduate school. Even if you do not plan to attend the same nursing school for a graduate degree, faculty change positions. It's not unreasonable to think that your paths will cross again.

Secondly, faculty can offer you a wealth of information about nursing practice, education, and research. They can offer guidance and share experiences with you about making decisions about your next step, whether it is applying for a position in clinical practice or applying to graduate school. What they have to offer is insight you may not be able to get anywhere else. *They've done it. They've been there.*

Thirdly, if you have a relationship with your professor, you are far more likely to be able to talk with you professor when you get a bad grade or circumstances arise that may affect performance. Professors may make exceptions and allowances given their understanding of the student's situation. This type of exchange would probably not happen if there was no relationship established.

Therefore, my suggestion for you to get the most out of nursing school is simple: *PLAN for your future. It is important to reflect about what it is you plan to do after nursing school and develop the relationships you think you will need to get there.* I know, when you are in nursing school, all you plan to do when you finish is to take the NCLEX and get a good job. Who is thinking about going back to school, right? But if you don't plan for the future, you may miss out on these great opportunities you can only get in nursing school.

Cynthia Ayres, PhD, RN
Assistant Professor, College of Nursing
Rutgers, The State University of New Jersey

References

Emailreplies.com. (n.d.). Retrieved November 1, 2007. from http://www.emailreplies.com/Index. html

Glater, J. (2006, February 21). To: Professor@University.edu Subject: Why it's all about me. *New York Times*, A1.

SEVEN

Getting the Most from Your Time in Class

Getting the Most from Your Classes Starts with Your Theory of Intelligence

Most of us have probably been impressed with someone else's intellectual achievement. Maybe this achievement was answering a difficult question in a class, doing especially well on an exam, or getting all of the questions on *Jeopardy* correct. The last time you witnessed someone doing something that was intellectually impressive, what did you to think about that person's intelligence? Would you characterize this person's intelligence as being fixed, which is similar to saying that intelligence is like height, and some people are tall while others are short people? Or would you characterize this person's intelligence as being malleable, which is similar to saying that intelligence is like muscle or lung capacity that can be developed with exercise? In other words, how do you think about intelligence?

Dr. Carol Dweck, a psychological researcher, has found that each of us has our own mindset or theory of intelligence and most people think of intelligence as being fixed or malleable. Those individuals who consider intelligence fixed, like height, have what she refers to as a *fixed mindset* or an *entity theory of intelligence.* Those individuals who consider intelligence malleable, like muscle or lung capacity, have a *growth mindset* or an *incremental theory of intelligence.*

Theories of Intelligence and Setting Goals

Why does having a specific mindset or theory of intelligence matter? Dr. Dweck and other researchers have found that what a student believes about intelligence and academic achievement influences how a student responds to the challenges and set-backs he or she will face during studies. Students who believe that intelligence is an unchangeable personal characteristic, an entity theory of intelligence, are less likely to develop academically because they avoid challenging themselves (Blackwell, Trzesnieweski, & Dweck, 2007). In contrast, students who believe that intelligence can be increased with effort, an incremental theory of intelligence, are more likely to engage in the challenging tasks that, while more risky, have the potential to increase academic competence. The evidence showing that a student's belief about intelligence influences academic achievement is strong. A number of researchers have found that, as compared to students who subscribed to the entity theory, students who were categorized as incremental theorists did better academically even after the researchers took into account, or controlled for, prior academic achievement (Blackwell et al., 2007; Henderson & Dweck, 1990).

Students who are entity theorists are more likely to adopt what are called *performance goals* and focus on validating their ability while at the same time avoiding any demonstration that they may lack ability (Good & Dweck, 2006). In contrast, students who are incremental theorists are more likely to pursue *learning goals.* Students pursuing learning goals are more likely than their classmates pursuing performance goals to apply their knowledge to a novel situation and process information at a deeper level (Good & Dweck, 2006). Moreover, incremental theorists are more likely than entity theorists to take on the challenges that lead to growth— growth in the classroom and growth outside the classroom.

You might be thinking, "I am an entity theorist. I have a fixed mindset. Am I doomed?" Fortunately, you can change your theory of intelligence. A number of studies show that academic achievement can be improved by teaching students about the incremental nature of intelligence (Aronson, Fried, & Good, 2002; Good, Aronson, & Inzlicht, 2003). For example, Aronson and colleagues studied college students who were randomly assigned to one of three groups. Each of the experimental groups received training on intelligence while the control group received no training during the semester. Students assigned to the incremental theory group received teaching on the incremental theory of intelligence and watched a film showing the way the brain forms new connections and "grows" every time new things are learned. Students assigned to the multiple intelligence group were taught that there are multiple types of intelligence and that individuals may be stronger in some areas than others. Each of the experimental groups also participated in a pen-pal program in which they wrote letters to junior high students discussing the perspective of intelligence emphasized in their group. The researchers found that the incremental theory group earned higher grade point averages (GPAs) and reported greater enjoyment of academics and greater valuing of academics than both the other groups.

Changing Your Mindset

Getting the most out of nursing school requires the right approach, and an important step toward having the right approach involves developing a growth mindset. In her book, *Mindset: The New Psychology of Success* (2006), Dweck provides suggestions for dealing with setbacks and challenges by changing one's mindset from a fixed mindset to a growth mindset, and in turn, improving one's success in school and life. In the discussion that follows, I adapt Dweck's suggestions to fit challenges and setbacks that one might encounter in nursing school.

Imagine you are halfway through your first semester of nursing school. By your own admission you are not off to a stellar start. You have received your midterm grades, and you are failing one course and barely passing the others. You need to make a comeback. How do you approach this challenge with a growth mindset?

Look at Your Goals

With a fixed mindset you might tell yourself "The nursing professors do not know how to teach," or "I am not smart enough for nursing school." These kinds of responses are not going to help you reach your goal of becoming a caring and competent nurse. You need to have a growth mindset that begins by looking at your goals and what is blocking them. What can you do to learn more? Are you working too many hours? Are you spending too much time in social pursuits? Have you used the recommendations in this book to organize your work habits and improve your learning? Think about the small-scale and large-scale changes you can make to help you achieve your goals.

Make a Concrete Plan

Developing better learning strategies or achieving any other goal requires making a plan that has the details of *when, where,* and *how.* So if your goal is to make more time for studying, you have to figure out *when* you are going to study (e.g., in the morning before class), *where* you are going to study (e.g., in the library), and *how* you are going to study (e.g., using the methods discussed in this book). These plans have to be more than empty promises to yourself. For example, if you are going to start studying in the morning before class, you are probably going to need to go to bed earlier. How can you make that happen? Do you spend less time watching television, fewer hours working, or what? For your plan to be successful you need the answers to these questions.

Feel Bad but Do Good

It does not feel good to come up short of any goal and, understandably, your mood will probably darken. An important element of a growth mindset is that you find a way to develop and implement a plan for the future despite feeling bad. If you are going to feel bad, you can sit and do nothing or you can take steps toward feeling better. You are better off in the long run by doing the latter.

Challenge Yourself

Developing a growth mindset begins with knowing that the more you challenge your mind to learn, the more your brain cells grow (Dweck, 2006). Your goal as a student in nursing school is not to show others (or yourself) how smart you are but to become a better and smarter nurse by pushing yourself to learn more.

Don't Run Away from Your Weaknesses

Challenging yourself begins with acknowledging that you have weaknesses and finding ways to develop your areas of weakness rather than relying solely on your strengths. You can see literal examples of individuals running away from their weaknesses on tennis courts every day. Many recreational tennis players (I am one of them) have a stronger backhand or stronger forehand stroke. Rather than returning a ball with their weaker stroke, they will "run around" their backhand or forehand and hit their stronger stroke. In the short-term they may win the point, but in the long term they have restricted their development as a tennis player. The same kind of avoidance happens in learning and restricts the development of students. Many students will "run around" subjects, classes, and situations that expose their weaknesses and try to use only their strengths. As with a tennis game, it may work for you in the short term, but it restricts growth. Get in the habit of forcing yourself to work on your weaknesses. For example, if you excel at writing papers but have trouble with oral presentations and you are enrolled in a course that gives you a choice, opt to make the oral presentation.

Real-World Snapshot 7-1

Begin to Know What You Don't Know Before Going to Class

In most classes students are assigned readings that are supposed to be completed before attending class. Students benefit from reading the material before going to class. It does not have to be an especially detailed reading, but it provides students with an understanding of what is going to be discussed in class and, more importantly, an understanding of what concepts are difficult to understand. In sum, students should know what questions they have or what they need to understand before they come to class, based on their readings, and they should listen for the answer or explanation and, if they don't hear it in the lecture, ask for it.

Randolph Rasch, PhD, RN
Professor and Director of the Family Nurse Practitioner Specialty
Vanderbilt University School of Nursing

Going to Class

It is no secret that at one time or another many students skip class. In fact, surveys show that 25–40% of college students report skipping class (Hurtado et al., 2007; Romer, 1993). The reasons some students offer for skipping class include lack of sleep, work due in other classes, and personal matters (e.g., funerals, illness). In contrast to students who miss class infrequently and skip class because of poor planning or personal issues, some students miss class on a regular basis and attend only to take exams and turn in assignments. Some of these chronic skippers report that they are not missing anything by skipping class because they can obtain notes of the class lectures online or from their peers, and they get all the information they need from assigned readings (Powers, 2007). These chronic skippers are not thinking ahead. While I acknowledge that unless class attendance is required to pass a class, some students (chronic skippers and occasional skippers) are able to pass courses without attending classes regularly, my recommendation is that you do not make a habit of missing nursing classes. In the section that follows, I offer evidence for why skipping class is not in your best interest.

Sidebar 7-1

The Importance of Attending Class

Occasionally, there are students who attend few, if any, classes for a particular course. They show up to take exams and leave afterwards. They feel that studying assigned readings is sufficient. And now that faculty often post outlines (such as Power Point slides) of their lectures on course Web sites (due to student expectation), the practice of skipping classes is becoming even more commonplace. This is because these students feel that they already have "the notes from class."

There are two reasons why skipping class is not a good idea. First, you will miss the professor's explanations and the emphasis of certain topics. You will miss examples or anecdotes that the professor uses to help you to understand the difficult content. You will miss the questions posed by your classmates, and the professor's answers of the topics covered in class. You will miss the essence of the professor-student and student-student interactions that promote learning in a way that cannot be duplicated in a book or a slide printout. Most importantly, you will miss the opportunity to interact with your professor and classmates. These are individuals you need to know in order to have a successful nursing school experience and the best outcomes. In a few short years, your classmates will be professional colleagues and your professor will be a valuable person with whom to network.

Second, whether or not faculty take attendance, you are not invisible and nameless. He or she will see your unfamiliar face during exams and think "Hmm, who is that? Oh, that's Mary Doe, she never comes to class. She only comes in for exams. She's not really interested in the course, she just wants to jump through a hoop."

Either way you have failed to create a favorable impression upon a faculty member you may need to call upon in the future. For example, you've applied for a summer job as a nursing extern and can't locate your clinical instructors to write a letter of recommendation for you. You need that letter desperately. Faculty who do not know you or do not have a favorable impression of you are unable to provide you with a good letter of recommendation. Keep this in mind throughout nursing school. Faculty are not obligated to write letters of recommendation for students. Think twice before sending out an angrily written e-mail after an exam.

Jeanne Ruggiero, PhD, RN, APN-C
Assistant Professor, College of Nursing
Seton Hall University

Real-World Snapshot 7-2

Tips for Students Who Are
Parents of Infants or Young Children

- Be realistic and do not try and finish everything in four years—I have seen too many students in a rush to get through nursing school as quickly as possible. They take a full load, and then they fail key courses. Then they register for another full load and fail more courses, and then they are out of the program. Look carefully at the school's requirements for course grades and GPA, and make sure you keep this in mind. Students are better off taking a lighter load and finishing everything in 5 years. Most nursing programs do not take students who have failed out of another nursing program.

- Go to a community college and take as many core courses (English, psychology, sociology, etc.), electives, and basic science courses (anatomy, physiology, chemistry, microbiology) as you can at that institution before matriculating into a 4-year nursing program—it is important to make sure that the courses will transfer (the core courses and sciences usually do). The advantage is these courses are less expensive. Take the pharmacology and pathophysiology courses in the nursing program because they may not transfer. As a rule, nursing courses do not transfer.

- When it is time to take the clinical courses, *take them alone*—This will allow you to focus on the clinical courses and get the most out of your nursing school education.

- Avoid accelerated programs—The students in these programs are so stressed out by the amount of material that they have to learn that they have no opportunity to synthesize the material and make sense of it. I think most students would be better off going to a regular program and taking the time required to study nursing.

Jeanne Ruggiero, PhD, RN, APN-C
Assistant Professor, College of Nursing
Seton Hall University

Better Grades

The primary reason for this recommendation is that there is strong evidence to suggest that students who attend class in college achieve higher GPAs (Devadoss & Foltz, 1996; Dolton, Marcenaro, & Navarro, 2003; Romer, 1993). Although your patients will be more concerned about the kind of care that you provide than the GPA you earned as a nursing student, and good grades do not necessarily indicate that you will be a good nurse, the best indicator of what you have learned in nursing school is your grades. Why is this the case? As discussed in Chapter 3, the outcome measure that all nursing schools use to evaluate student achievement and ability to practice competently is the National Council Licensure Examination (NCLEX-RN), and there is strong evidence that students who pass the NCLEX-RN have significantly higher GPAs than those students who fail (Beeson & Kissling, 2001; Daley, Kirkpatrick, Frazier, Chung, & Moser, 2003; Endres, 1997; Roncoli, Lisanti, & Falcone, 2000).

Real-World Snapshot 7-3

Don't Drive Yourself Crazy About Grades

In nursing school it is easy to get wrapped up in grades, and some students drive themselves crazy trying to get all *A*'s. Although good grades are important, students should keep in mind that an occasional *B does not* doom your chances of getting into graduate school, *does not* mean that you will not be able to get a good job as a nurse, and *does not* mean that you did not learn as much as a student in the class who got a *B*⁺ or an *A*. Devote the energy you might waste on obsessing about grades to learning as much as you can.

Joy Atkins, MA, RN
Adjunct Instructor, Department of Nursing
Rutgers, The State University of New Jersey

Sidebar 7-2

Reach Out to Your Professor

It means a lot to me when students who have done poorly on an exam or an assignment take the time to let me know that they are concerned about not doing well and ask me for my advice on how to do better.

Jeanne Ruggiero, PhD, RN, APN-C
Assistant Professor, College of Nursing
Seton Hall University

More Options in the Future

In addition to the association between class attendance, GPA, and NCLEX pass rates, there is an association between GPA and your options after nursing school. Many readers of this book want to gain admission to RN to BSN programs after nursing school or gain admission into graduate degree programs. Having sat on many admission committees for undergraduate and graduate programs, I know firsthand that an applicant's GPA in nursing school influences admission decisions. Graduate admissions committees know that students who did well as undergraduates are likely to do well in graduate schools. Moreover, there is some evidence that employers weigh GPAs heavily in making hiring decisions, and many will not look at candidates with GPAs lower than 3.0 (Koeppel, 2006). The severity of the current nursing shortage makes it unlikely that GPAs will influence the hiring decisions of potential employers in the near future, but there have been surpluses of nurses before, and there probably will be again.

Reading in Nursing School

In an ideal world all of us would be able to open a book, read the words, and retain all the information. Unfortunately, very few of us (if any of us) have a photographic memory; thus we cannot retain and recall words and ideas that we have read only once maybe hours, days, or years earlier. When you read material that interests you (e.g., reading with a purpose) or material you are familiar with, you have a much easier time storing that information to use later. One reason for this is that when you read something you truly want to understand, you try harder. For example, if I were shipwrecked on a deserted island and the one thing that washed up on the island was the book *Surviving on a Deserted Island for Dummies,* I would read and seek to comprehend every word in that book—my life would depend on it.

In addition to reading with a purpose, the other factor that influences your understanding and retention of material you read is what you do with the information after you read it. Research on reading suggests that retention is enhanced when you use the ideas or concepts that you have read. It is more likely that I would retain information on building a fire on a deserted island if I read the chapter discussing that skill and then built a fire, than if I read the chapter on building a fire and then went fishing and took a nap.

Improving Your Ability to Retain Information Through SQ3R

Thankfully there are other ways to improve your ability to comprehend and retain information that do not require being shipwrecked. One popular method is known as the SQ3R study method. The letters SQ3R stand for *survey, question, read, recite,* and *review,* and refer to a study method that was developed in the 1940s by Frank Robinson, an Ohio State University psychologist. Since its inception this method has been used by college students to improve their ability to comprehend and retain information. The beauty of this method is that, if followed, it forces one to read actively and systematically. Reading in this manner increases the likelihood that the time one spends will result in the retention of information.

Most students read a textbook chapter like they would mow a lawn—relatively mindlessly. A better approach to reading a textbook or other academic material is to treat the activity like tending a garden rather than mowing a lawn. A gardener surveys the garden (the Survey step in SQ3R) and decides what he or she wants to accomplish (the Question step in SQ3R): pick some ripe tomatoes, weed, plant, or what? The gardener then works to accomplish the goals (the Read step in SQ3R) he or she has set. In contrast to mowing the lawn, this activity is far from mindless; the gardener is constantly assessing progress (the Recitation step in SQ3R) that has been made toward accomplishing the goal. Finally, the gardener evaluates (the Review step in SQ3R) what has been achieved.

To get the most out of the time you spend on a reading assignment it is crucial that you read systematically. Whether you choose to use the SQ3R system, adapt the SQ3R, or come up with your own system doesn't matter—as long as you have a system. The following sections describe in detail how to use the SQ3R system.

Survey

As discussed, the first step of SQ3R is to survey. The survey step involves looking at the entire reading assignment. Your goal in surveying the reading assignment is to figure out where to put your emphasis. Certain sections will be more important than others. You will answer the following questions in this step:

1. What is covered in this chapter?
2. What am I expecting to learn in this chapter?
3. What do I already know about what is covered in this chapter from my previous coursework, present coursework, life experiences, and so on?

After you answer these questions, you are ready to quickly skim the reading assignment. During your skim of the chapter, make a mental note of the main ideas contained within the chapter, read the headings, inspect the graphs and tables, and look at the pictures. End the survey step by reading the summary of the chapter that is usually provided. You now know the major points that are contained in the chapter.

Question

Now that you have surveyed the chapter and you have a pretty good idea of what you should be getting out of the reading, turn back to the beginning of the chapter. Look at the headings and subheadings again because, you know from your experience and education, each of these headings reflects the central ideas for the paragraphs that follow. In the question step of SQ3R you will turn each of the headings or subheadings into a question. For example, imagine that you have been assigned the chapter on respiratory physiology to read in your physiology textbook. Using SQ3R to prepare yourself to read actively, you notice the heading "Effect of Ph and Temperature on Oxygen Transport." Turn that heading into a question before you begin reading the paragraphs that follow. You could transpose this heading into a question any number of ways: What is the effect of pH on temperature and oxygen transport? Or how are temperature and oxygen transport influenced by pH? What is most important is that you frame the question so that you are seeking to answer questions that relate to your overall goals for the reading assignment.

Read

You have completed the survey and question steps of SQ3R; now you are reading to focus on the main idea of the section. In your first reading you are not going to let yourself get bogged down or distracted by the minor details of the section; instead you are focusing on the "big picture" and concentrating only on the details that support the main idea. If the minor details are important for the overall goals of your reading assignment, you can focus on those elements in a second or third reading. *After* you have finished reading the section (*not* while you are reading the section), identify the main points and key terms by underlining or using a yellow highlighter (yellow highlights are supposed to improve recall). Many students find that writing their notes in a separate notebook or into a word-processing document on the computer is extremely useful. In fact, there is some evidence that the physical act of writing improves the retention of information (Parker & Goodkin, 1987).

Recite

Recitation is the second R in SQ3R, and it involves a self-assessment of mastery of the content in the section of text that has just been read. To assess your mastery of the content, determine whether you can summarize the most important ideas in the section in your own words. The recitation phase of SQ3R involves explaining the material back to yourself aloud. Do you know what the big picture is? Refer back to the questions that you developed prior to reading the section; are you able to answer those questions? For example, if you read the section on "Effect of Ph and Temperature on Oxygen Transport" in your physiology textbook, you should know that the tissues receive more oxygen when the blood pH drops (Bohr effect) and when the temperature rises. As a nurse the big picture is that a lower pH in the blood is suggestive of an increased carbon dioxide concentration that is indicative of a more active tissue that requires more oxygen. If you have not mastered the material, read the section again. An advantage of keeping a notebook or a Word file open while you read is that you can write a question to test your mastery of the material. Such questions might look like this:

- Physical activity has which of the following effects on Ph and temperature:
  - Raises the temperature and lowers the Ph
  - Raises the temperature and raises the Ph
  - Lowers the temperature and lowers the Ph
  - Lowers the temperature and raises the Ph

After you have mastered the material, move to the next section of your reading, applying the question-read-recite process.

Review

To complete the final step—review—look at your reading assignment and the notes that you kept, and summarize the main ideas. Your recall of some of the concepts and ideas may be a little fuzzy; take time to sharpen your understanding in those areas. If you have been thorough in completing the other steps of SQ3R, the review step can be completed fairly quickly. Depending on how well you do at retaining information over the long term, you will need periodic reviews of your reading assignment and notes on a daily or weekly basis. See what works best for you. If you find that the information is taking a while to come back to you, shorten the period of time between review sessions.

Summary

The SQ3R system can sound like a substantial amount of work, and it is; however, keep two points in mind. First, and most important, in nursing school you are preparing to promote, maintain, and restore the health and well-being of others. This is a great responsibility, and it requires sacrifice on your part. Second, while SQ3R is intensive and time consuming in the short term, in the long term you are more time efficient than you would be if you are not systematic in your approach to reading. If you are going to invest time out of your day for class readings, make your investment count. Simply turning pages is not enough. SQ3R can assist you in making the most out of the time you spend reading for class.

Appendix 7-1 provides a demonstration of SQ3R using sample reading material from a nursing textbook.

Taking Notes in Class and Lecture

Most professors use lectures to discuss the central concepts of the class, emphasizing the material that they believe to be most salient for your nursing practice (consequently, most likely to be on the exam). Lectures provide students with an opportunity to sync their studying with the professor's emphasis. Although most students know that it is important to retain the information from class and lectures, research on learning and memory suggests that most individuals are able to retain only a fraction of what is discussed during a lecture. Consequently, to get the most out of lectures and class discussion, one needs to do more than go to class and take a seat. Discussed in this section are some general and specific approaches to note taking and actively listening to get the most out of class time.

There are good reasons for taking notes in class. Kiewra (1985b) found that, even when students do not review notes, the students who took notes performed at higher levels than those who did not take notes. This finding suggests that the physical process of recording notes is important, because students must process the information to write it down, which helps with retention and recall. In fact, while students have about a 50% chance of recalling noted information on a test, they have only about a 15% chance of recalling nonnoted information (Aiken, Thomas, & Shennum, 1975). Unfortunately, the notes of most students are woefully incomplete and capture only 20–40% of the important ideas presented in a lecture (Kiewra, 1985b; O'Donnell & Dansereau, 1993). The following recommendations are included to improve your note taking:

- Be prepared—Read the assignments before coming to class. Your note taking will improve by coming to class prepared because you will already have a sense of where the class discussion is likely to be heading.
- Don't try to save paper—Keep your notes in a large notebook; preferably a three-ring binder. Write only on one side of the paper and leave plenty of space in your notes so that you can expand on and add to points as the lecture progresses. Keep a separate binder for each class.

- Use a note-taking system—Use an established note-taking system or develop one of your own. The best systems are in outline form or have a numbering system that distinguishes main points from minor points that follow. In addition, abbreviate whenever possible. Start using the abbreviations that you will use as a nurse. See Box 7-1 for a list of abbreviations that you should use. In Box 7-2 is a list of error-prone abbreviations that you *should not use* because they have been found to be associated with medication errors (Institute for Safe Medication Practices, 2007).

- Keep taking notes—Many professors will provide complete or skeletal notes of their lectures. While there is strong evidence to show that complete and skeletal notes enhance learning, continue to take notes on the space provided of these notes, in the margins, or in a notebook for later review. As noted, there is value in the process of taking notes (it increases focus); so even if your professor has given you notes, keep taking notes of your own. Taking notes helps you keep your mind on the lesson at hand. There is a direct association between the quantity of notes a student takes and achievement (Kiewra & Fletcher, 1984; Kiewra, 2002).

- Follow the cues—The quantity of notes may be related to performance, but your goal is not to write down every word uttered by your professor—that would be difficult and a poor use of your class time. The process of thinking about what you are copying into your notes is why note taking improves retention and recall. You may be wondering what to write down. Most professors think that everything they say in class (and out of class) is noteworthy, but you can usually figure out from the cues provided by your professor what he or she believes to be especially important. Cues include: (1) content that he or she has taken the time to put on the blackboard, whiteboard, or highlighted in a PowerPoint slide; (2) content that he or she has repeated a couple of times with emphasis; (3) content that he or she has summarized at the end of class or reviewed at the beginning of class, and (4) formulas, definitions, and specific facts. Include this type of content in your notes, and make a point of highlighting it.

- Do it right the first time—If you write legibly so you can read what you write, you won't have to recopy your notes. It is all right to print, and there are some modified writing styles that enhance legibility. Many students do recopy their notes, but your time is better spent reviewing your notes and adding to what you have already written than rewriting your notes.

Box 7-1   Nursing Abbreviations and Symbols

a	before	JVP	jugular venous pressure
ABD	abdomen	KVO	keep vein open
ABG	arterial blood gas	lb	pound
AC	before eating	LLQ	left lower quadrant
ADL	activities of daily living	MI	myocardial infarction
AGA	appropriate for gestational age	MVA	motor vehicle accident
AIDS	acquired immune deficiency syndrome	neg	negative
		NKA	no known allergies
AM	morning	NPO	nothing by mouth
AP	anteroposterior	NSAID	nonsteroidal anti-inflammatory drugs
B/K	below knee	NV	nausea and vomiting
BID	twice a day	O_2	oxygen
BILAT	bilateral	OD	overdose or right eye
BM	bowel movement		
BP	blood pressure	OS	left eye
BS	bowel or breath sounds	OU	both eyes
BW	body weight	p	after
c	with	PI	present illness
CABG	coronary artery bypass graft	PM	after noon
CSF	cerebrospinal fluid	po	(per os) by mouth
CVA	cerebral vascular accident	prn	when necessary
CXR	chest x-ray	pt	patient
DC	discontinue/discharge	Q	every
DX	diagnosis	RLQ	right lower quadrant
EENT	eye, ear, nose, and throat	RX	prescription
ETOH	ethanol/alcohol	s	without
FTT	failure to thrive	SOB	short of breath
FX	fracture	SX	symptoms
GI	gastrointestinal	TID	three times a day
GU	genitourinary	TX	treatment
H_2O	water	URI	upper respiratory infection
HA	headache	VSS	vital signs stable
HGB	hemoglobin	W/U	workup
HS	at bedtime	x	times
HTN	hypertension	YTD	year to date
HX	history	♀	female
IBW	ideal body weight	♂	male
IM	intramuscular	↑	increase
IV	intravenous	↓	decrease

Box 7-2 Abbreviations Not to Use from the Official "Do Not Use" List

U	unit	Write "unit"
IU	International Unit	Write "International Unit"
Q.D.	every day, daily	Write "daily"
Trailing zero X.0 mg		Write "X mg"
.X		Write "0.X mg"
MS	morphine sulfate or	Write "morphine sulfate"
	magnesium sulfate	Write "magnesium sulfate"
>	greater than	Write "greater than"
<	less than	Write "less than"
Abbreviations for drug names		Write drug names in full
Apothecary units		Use metric units
@		Write "at"
cc		Write "ml" or "milliliters"
μg		Write "mcg" or "micrograms"

■ Develop your focus—Listening to an academic lecture is usually not entertaining like a comedy show or a poetry reading. Consequently, to process the information you are taking into your notes, you need to focus. Tips to improve your focus include the following:
  • Look at the speaker during the lecture. Nonverbal cues are being transmitted by the speaker that you might miss if you have your head buried in your notes.
  • Focus on the content of what is being said rather than the delivery. If you are recording the number of times the speaker says "you know" or scratches his or her ear during the lecture, you are focusing on delivery and missing content.
  • Keep your focus clear by asking yourself questions during the lecture such as: What key points are being made by the speaker? How does this fit with what I know from previous lectures? How is this lecture organized?
  • Sit in the front of the class. Many students avoid sitting in the front of the class. If you sit as close to the front of the class as possible, you will have fewer distractions (the attractive classmate, the dozing classmate, etc.).
■ No tape recording—Although there are probably some students who benefit from tape recording lectures, for most students, tape recording class lectures is not an efficient alternative, or a good complement, to note taking.

In addition to the hassles of keeping track of tapes, getting the professor's permission to record a lecture, and worrying about running out of tape or batteries, a tape-recorded lecture still has to be listened to actively at some point. This means that you have to find the time and place to pay attention to this content. Listening to a tape-recorded lecture while you are exercising or driving in your car means that you are not giving your full attention to the lecture. You will benefit more by developing your note-taking abilities and spending your time reviewing the lecture than listening to the lecture in class and outside of class.

Learn to Speak the Language

A substantial portion of your education in nursing school involves introducing you to the language of nursing, science, and health care. As with most other disciplines or professions (e.g., engineering, military, culinary arts), nursing and health care have their own language, and to be a part of that discipline you have to speak the language. For example, most nurses in the United States would understand the following phrase: "I have an order to give the Vitamin H po at HS and IM prn," to mean that the patient is to receive Haldol (antipsychotic medication) by mouth at bedtime and by injection when needed.

To get the most out of your classes, you also have to learn to speak the language of that content area. Without the language of these content areas, you will not be able to grasp the larger concepts. Why is language so fundamental to learning? One hypothesis is that language is required for higher-level thinking and shapes how one understands the world (Monroe & Orme, 2002). Consequently, in your studying and note taking, focus on understanding the meaning of the words used. Get out of the habit of glossing over words that are unfamiliar. For example, take the following sentence, which is typical of pathophysiology textbooks:

> Unlike **somatic neurons,** which conduct impulses along a single axon from the spinal cord to the neuromuscular junction, **autonomic motor control** involves two neurons in the **efferent pathway.**

Take the time to open up a dictionary or thesaurus; check in the glossary of the book or a previous page as to what is meant by somatic neurons, autonomic motor control, and efferent pathway. Draw a diagram or make a note to remind yourself that *efferent* refers to the transport of something away from a central location and *afferent* refers to the transport of something toward a center. Of course, in the short term, taking time out to understand the terminology will slow you down; however, in the long term you will get more out of your studies.

Class Participation

In many nursing classes a portion of your grade (10–15% is typical) will be based upon class participation. Class participation is important for several reasons. First, your comments provide your professor an opportunity to determine whether you are grasping the concepts that are being discussed, which, in turn, allows your professor to target his or her presentation more effectively. Second, class participation can enliven the class and break the monotony. As discussed in the chapter on oral presentation, developing a dialogue with your audience makes it more interesting for the audience and more interesting for you as the speaker. Third, speaking in class allows you to practice the skills you need to become an effective public speaker. In your career as a healthcare professional, it is likely that you will attend conferences and public meetings where the ability to be persuasive or to ask a well-thought question will be important.

Your professor's evaluation of your class participation is based more on the quality of your participation than the quantity. It is not how often you speak in class but the value of what you have to offer. Valuable contributions are those questions and comments that add to the learning environment. Imagine in your pediatric theory course your professor is discussing the nurse's role in educating parents on establishing rules and guidelines for children's behavior, or *limit setting*. As part of this topic your professor discusses some of the more common strategies of dealing with toddler and child misbehavior (e.g., corporal punishment, reasoning and scolding, ignoring, and time-outs) and asks your class to comment on these strategies.

Below is an example of what an outstanding contribution from a student might sound like:

> I was occasionally spanked as a child, and, while I didn't like it, I do not think that there were any lasting ill effects. However, I know from reading that I have done that the topic of spanking and corporal punishment is controversial. For example, the American Academy of Pediatrics and other child development experts have reported that in certain circumstances the use of corporal punishment is

an effective form of child discipline. In contrast, in a study that appeared in the July 2002 issue of the *Psychological Bulletin*, the author analyzed 88 studies and found a significant association between nonabusive spanking during childhood and negative developmental outcomes (Gershoff, 2002). Consequently, I think in our education to parents we should err on the side of being overcautious and discourage spanking.

What makes this contribution so outstanding? First, the student provides strong evidence to back up her opinion that nurses should discourage parents from spanking their children by referring to an article that she read in the *Psychological Bulletin*, a peer-reviewed journal. Peer-reviewed journals are published on a monthly or quarterly basis; however, instead of names like *Sports Illustrated* and *Time*, they have titles like *Child Development*, the *Journal of Research on Adolescence*, and *Death Studies*. Researchers submit manuscripts or papers to these journals to be reviewed by experts in the field. The researchers who submit the manuscripts and the reviewers are anonymous to each other. The reviewers critique the strengths and weaknesses of the research papers, and based on this critique an editor of the journal decides to either reject the paper or have the author of the paper revise it based on the reviewers' comments. After revisions are made, the researcher will resubmit the paper for another round of critiques. This round of critiques may result in a rejection, more revisions by the author, or acceptance of the paper for publication.

What else makes this contribution outstanding? The student makes a coherent and persuasive argument by acknowledging that she had been spanked. She then moves beyond her personal experiences and expands her comment into the scientific domain by comparing and contrasting the opinions of child development experts. Moreover, the content of this student's remarks suggests that the student did more than the assigned reading from the textbook to prepare for class. Finally, this student's contribution is outstanding because it opens the door for an interesting dialogue to develop in class on corporal punishment and the nurse's role in educating parents.

Below is an example of an adequate contribution:

The reading in the textbook mentioned that one of the problems with spanking is that children may become "used to getting hit," and the parent may have to hit the child harder or with other objects like belts or paddles to get the same effect. I don't think that most parents want to inflict pain on their kids, so I think in my teaching to parents on discipline I would recommend that they use time-outs to discipline their child.

What makes this contribution adequate? The strengths of this contribution are that it is clear that the student prepared for class by completing the assigned reading. Moreover, the student used the reading to provide a logical rationale for why he would encourage a parent to employ time-outs to discipline their child rather than spanking. This contribution opens the door to more in-class dialogue, but it is unlikely that this contribution would generate the range of dialogue that the outstanding contribution would generate.

Below are some examples of inappropriate or unsatisfactory contributions:

Uuuhhh...

Do we need to know this for the test?

Everybody knows that spanking a child is good/bad and children who are spanked grow up to be good citizens/criminals. As a child I was spanked/ not spanked, and I turned out fine.

As discussed above, the quality of your contribution matters more than the frequency of participation; however, just showing up for class is probably not enough to receive credit for class participation. One has to provide contributions that enhance the discussion in class or at least demonstrate to your professor that you have prepared for class.

While one student's failure to participate in class discussions does not enhance class discussions and will probably earn that student a poor grade for class participation, contributing comments like the second and third examples detract from the learning environment and are almost sure to doom a student's grade for participation. Consider the question, "Do we need to know this for the test?" Unfortunately, this question has been asked too often in both the nursing classes I teach and the classes I attended as a student in nursing school. This type of question, if it needs to be asked, should not be asked during class. The student who poses this question appears to be more interested in performance on a test than in developing the knowledge he or she will need to promote the health and well-being of future patients. Such a comment distracts the professor and the class from the opportunity to discuss something important and enriching.

Regarding the third example, while this contribution does relate to the current topic and it is not disrespectful of anyone's race or religion, it is hard to imagine that the class would not be better off without this type of dialogue injected into the classroom environment. The insights provided in this contribution are anecdotal and do not reflect a review of the science on child development. There may be value in using one's experiences as a starting point; however, it is important to move beyond personal experiences and anecdotes. These kinds of anecdotes and types of expression (e.g., "everybody knows") are fine for radio call-in shows where they need to fill up airtime, but they do not fit the goals for class participation. The goal of participation in nursing school discussions is to enhance and expand knowledge and understanding around topics that will be important in the lives of the patients you will work with as a nurse.

Sidebar 7-3

For Students Who Fail

In most nursing programs, students who fail to receive a passing grade in a nursing course have to "sit out" and wait for the nursing course they failed to be offered again. This is a frustrating and stressful situation; however, it is important that students take the time to consider why they failed. Did the student fail to give nursing school a high enough priority? Was it poor study skills? Was it the case that the student was working too many hours? Whatever the reason, the student needs to give serious thought to correcting this situation before retaking the failed course. For example, if a student worked too many hours, the student should plan on working fewer or no hours the next time he or she takes the course they failed. However, if in addition to nursing studies the student was a parent of young children, the student may want to think about waiting 2 years until the child (or children) is a little older before returning to their nursing studies.

Jane Kurz, PhD, RN
Associate Professor, Department of Nursing
Temple University

References

Aiken, E. G., Thomas, G. S., & Shennum, W. A. (1975). Memory for a lecture: Effects of notes, lecture rate and informational density. *Journal of Educational Psychology, 67,* 439–444.

Aronson, J., Fried, C. B., & Good, C. (2002). Reducing stereotype threat and boosting academic achievement of African-American students: The role of conceptions of intelligence. *Journal of Experimental Social Psychology, 38,* 113–125.

Beeson, S. A. & Kissling, G. (2001). Predicting success for baccalaureate graduates on the NCLEX-RN. *Journal of Professional Nursing, 17,* 121–127.

Blackwell, L., Trzesniewski, K., & Dweck, C. S. (2007). Implicit theories of intelligence predict achievement across an adolescent transition: A longitudinal study and an intervention. *Child Development, 78,* 246–263.

Daley, L. K., Kirkpatrick, B. L., Frazier, S. K., Chung, M. L. & Moser, D. K. (2003). Predictors of NCLEX-RN success in a baccalaureate nursing program as a foundation for remediation. *Journal of Nursing Education, 42,* 390–398.

Devadoss, S., & Foltz, J. (1996). Evaluation of factors influencing student class attendance and performance. *American Journal of Agricultural Economics, 78,* 499–507.

Dolton, P., Marcenaro, O. D., & Navarro, L. (2003). The effective use of student time: A stochastic frontier production function case study. *Economics of Education Review, 22,* 547–560.

Dweck, C. S. (2006). *Mindset: The new psychology of success.* Random House: New York.

Endres, D. (1997). A comparison of predictors of success on NCLEX-RN for African American, foreign-born, and white baccalaureate graduates. *Journal of Nursing Education, 36,* 365–371.

Gershoff, E. T. (2002). Corporal punishment by parents and associated child behaviors and experiences: A meta-analytic and theoretical review. *Psychological Bulletin, 128,* 539–579.

Good, C., Aronson, J., & Inzlicht, M. (2003). Improving adolescents' standardized test performance: An intervention to reduce the effects of stereotype threat. *Journal of Applied Developmental Psychology, 24,* 645–662.

Good, C., and Dweck, C. S. (2006). A motivational approach to reasoning, resilience and responsibility. In R. J. Sternberg & R. F. Subotnik (Eds.), *Optimizing student success in school with the other three Rs: Reasoning, resilience, and responsibility* (pp. 39–55). Charlotte, NC: Information Age Publishing, Inc.

Henderson, V. L. & Dweck, C. S. (1990). Motivation and achievement. In S. S. Feldman & G. R. Elliot (Eds.), *At the threshold: The developing adolescent* (pp. 308–329). Cambridge, MA: Harvard University Press.

Hurtado, S., Sax, L. J., Saenz, V., Harper, C. E., Oseguera, L., Curley, J., et al. (2007). Findings from the 2005 administration of your first college year YFCY: National Aggregates. *Higher Education Research Institute. University of California Los Angeles.* Retrieved May 26, 2007, from http://www.gseis.ucla.edu/heri/PDFs/2005_YFCY_REPORT_FINAL.pdf.

Institute for Safe Medication Practices. (2007). *ISMP and FDA campaign to eliminate use of error-prone abbreviations.* Retrieved October 1, 2007, from http://www.ismp.org/tools/abbreviations

Kiewra, K. A. (1985b). Students' note-taking behaviors and the efficacy of providing the instructor's notes for review. *Contemporary Educational Psychology, 10,* 378–386.

Kiewra, K. (2002). How classroom teachers can help students learn and teach them how to learn. *Theory Into Practice, 41,* 71–80.

Kiewra, K. A., & Fletcher, H. J. (1984). The relationship between levels of note taking and achievement. *Human Learning, 3,* 273–280.

Koeppel, D. (2006, December 31). Those low grades in college may haunt your job search. *New York Times,* A1.

Monroe, E. E., & Orme, M. P. (2002). Developing mathematical vocabulary. *Preventing School Failure, 46,* 139–142.

O'Donnell, A., & Dansereau, D. F. (1993). Learning from lectures: Effects of cooperative review. *Journal of Experimental Education, 61,* 116–125.

Parker, R. P., & Goodkin, V. (1987). *The consequences of writing: Enhancing learning in the disciplines.* Upper Montclair, NJ: Boynton/Cook.

Powers, E. (2007). Elephant not in the room. *Inside Higher Ed.com.* Retrieved May 26, 2007, from http://insidehighered.com/news/2007/05/01/absent.

Romer, D. (1993). "Do students go to class? Should they?" *Journal of Economic Perspectives, 7,* 167–174.

Roncoli, M., Lisanti, P., & Falcone, A. (2000). Characteristics of baccalaureate graduates and NCLEX-RN performance. *Journal of the New York State Nurses Association, 31,* 17–19.

APPENDIX 7-A

Active Reading with SQ3R

Steps

In the discussion below, text (beginning on page 112) from a nursing textbook is used to provide an example of how SQ3R is used to actively read.

Survey

The section of reading comes from a chapter titled "Review of the Aging of Physiological Systems." Before reading the assigned section, you may want to think about what you hope to know after reading the chapter. In many textbooks, the authors provide a list of learning objectives for students at the beginning of each chapter. The authors of this chapter have provided six learning objectives that are listed at the beginning of the chapter that the reader should accomplish after completing the chapter:

The reader will be able to:

1. Describe the aging process of each physiological system.
2. Distinguish between aging and age-related disease.
3. Describe how the aging process of each physiological system correlates with the functional ability of the older adult.
4. Explain how the aging process of one system interacts with and/or affects other physiological systems.

5. Acknowledge that not every aspect of every physiological system changes with age.
6. Recognize that aging changes are partially dependent upon an individual's health behaviors and preventive health measures.

Give some thought to how the learning objectives of the authors compare with your learning objectives. Remember that just because content is provided in your assigned reading does not mean that it is relevant to what you need to know as a student. Think about how the assigned reading fits within the course.

As part of your survey of the assigned reading, you also want to spend some time looking at the headings to get a sense of what is covered. This is also the time to look at the figures and any graphs. Try to make sense of what is being presented as best you can. Think about how it fits with what you may have learned in a previous class. For example, you probably covered some of the content on the muscular system in your anatomy and physiology course.

Question

Your next step in SQ3R is to turn the headings into questions. For example, the first heading is "Skeletal Muscle: Structure and Function." Depending on what your learning objectives are for the course, you might change this into the questions: How are skeletal muscles structured? How do skeletal muscles function? As you read the assigned reading (next step in SQ3R), you want to answer these questions. The importance of reading with a purpose cannot be overemphasized. Your purpose in reading is not merely to complete the reading but to have your questions answered. When you get to the reading component of SQ3R, you will be constantly referring back to your questions as you read each section. Anytime you find yourself drifting or not reading actively, refocus your thinking by referring to your questions.

Reading

As discussed earlier in the section on SQ3R, you are probably going to need to read your assigned reading at least twice to get the most out of it. In your first reading you are just going for an overview, focusing on the main points of the assignment, and answering the questions that you developed from the headings and subheadings. For example, look at the section "Skeletal Muscle: Structure and Function." As you read this the first time, focus on those sentences that answer the questions: How are skeletal muscles structured? How do skeletal muscles function? By reading the first paragraph of the section and the first two sentences of the second paragraph, you should be able to answer the first question. To answer the second question you can skim the first few sentences of the second paragraph until you get to the sentence, "Muscle contraction results when actin molecules are pulled toward the center of the sarcomere in a ratcheting motion."

Depending on what your goals are for the reading, on your second reading you might want to include in your notes definitions for the terms that are styled bold in the text: **myofibrils, actins, myosins, sacromeres,** and explain how they contribute to the function of skeletal muscle. On the other hand, after reading this section once and answering your questions, you might decide that this content is not that relevant to your learning goals and not worth reading a second time and taking notes. How much emphasis you place on a section of a reading assignment is determined by the goals that you established in your initial survey.

As discussed earlier, part of your goal as a student is to determine which areas of the reading are most important to focus on. If you are fortunate, you may have a professor in nursing school who will be very specific in the readings assigned; however, most professors do not have the time or inclination to sort through each chapter in a textbook and identify the areas you need to focus on and the areas that are not relevant to the class. Consequently, you have to make that determination on your own from the syllabus, class lectures, clinical experiences, and your own interests as a nursing student. For example, the section on muscles includes a long paragraph on the two distinct physiological types of muscle fibers—fast twitch and slow twitch— which may be irrelevant to what your learning goals are in the course but may be of interest to you because you are interested in the science of exercise.

Recitation

Imagine that the section on muscle structure and function is important, and you have typed notes directly into a word-processing document, written notes out longhand into a notebook where you keep your notes from the reading, or written the notes directly onto note cards that you plan to study from. In the recitation step of the SQ3R process, you recite aloud what you have learned from the reading. For example, you should be able to answer in your own words how skeletal muscles function: "Skeletal muscles contract. This contraction occurs when the actin molecules are pulled toward the center of the sarcomere."

During the recitation process you can also develop questions to test yourself on the reading assignment. For example, The myofibrils of skeletal muscles contain two types of protein molecules. They are _____ and _____. The answers are actins and myosins. Another example would be: What is sarcopenia? The answer is it is the age-related (versus disease or starvation related) reduction in muscle mass that occurs in all elderly persons.

As discussed earlier, your goal through recitation is to transfer the information from your short-term memory into your long-term memory. When you are able to explain what you read back to yourself, it is likely that you are approaching or have attained that goal. Once you are there, you can move into the final step of the SQ3R process—review.

Review

This step gets repeated every day or every couple of days depending on how well you can demonstrate mastery of the material to yourself. You demonstrate mastery by taking out your notes and reciting aloud the content or answering the questions that you developed. When you have mastered the material, you should be able to quickly retrieve the material from your memory and explain the concept, term, or idea back to yourself accurately or answer the question with little or no hesitation.

1. Describe the aging process of each physiological system.
2. Distinguish between aging and age-related disease.
3. Describe how the aging process of each physiological system correlates with the functional ability of the older adult.
4. Explain how the aging process of one system interacts with and/or affects other physiological systems.
5. Acknowledge that not every aspect of every physiological system changes with age.
6. Recognize that aging changes are partially dependent upon an individual's health behaviors and preventive health measures.

Excerpt from "Review of the Aging of Physiological Systems"

The Muscle

The body's muscular system is composed of three types of muscle—skeletal muscle, smooth muscle, and cardiac muscle. Skeletal muscles, examples of which include the bicep, tricep, quadricep, hamstring, and gastrocnemius (calf) muscle, make up the majority of the body's overall muscle mass. Skeletal muscle is also the muscle type in which most age-related changes occur. Thus, skeletal muscle and its changes with age will be the focus of our discussion about the aging muscle.

Skeletal Muscle: Structure and Function

Skeletal muscles are composed of several thin muscle bundles. These bundles are held together with connective tissue but are able to move independently of one another (Arking, 1998). The muscle bundles are composed of several muscle fibers, each of which is formed from the fusion of numerous individual myofibrils.

Myofibrils contain two types of protein molecules—**actins** and **myosins**. Actin and myosin molecules are arranged in a parallel, overlapping manner within compartments called **sarcomeres**. The overlap of actin and myosin within the sarcomere results in a pattern of alternating light and dark bands, which accounts for the striated, or striped, appearance of skeletal muscle. In a state of rest, actin molecules overlap both ends of the myosin molecules, which are centered within the sarcomere. Muscle contraction results when actin molecules are pulled toward the center of the sarcomere in a ratcheting motion. This contraction of skeletal muscle is controlled by an individual's own volition; hence, skeletal muscle has also been termed voluntary muscle.

Although muscle fibers have a common basic structure, they can be divided into two distinct physiological types, fast-twitch and slow-twitch fibers. These two fiber types produce the same amount of force per contraction; however, they produce this force at different rates. White fast-twitch fibers contract quickly and provide short bursts of energy, but they fatigue quickly. As a result of these contractile properties, fast-twitch fibers are generally used for high-intensity, low-endurance, generally anaerobic activities such as sprinting and weight lifting. Red slow-twitch fibers contract slowly but steadily and are not easily fatigued. Therefore, these fibers are best suited for use in aerobic activities of low intensity but high endurance, such as long-distance running. Slow-twitch fibers are also used for postural activities, such as the supporting of the head by the neck. Every person is born with a fixed ratio of fast-twitch to slow-twitch muscle fibers. However, the ratio may vary from one body location to another, and one person may have a greater ratio of fast-twitch to slow-twitch fibers in a particular location than does another person. This phenomenon is part of what can result in one individual being, for example, a better sprinter or better long-distance runner than another.

Aging of the Skeletal Muscle

Sarcopenia

A reduction in muscle mass occurs to at least some degree in all elderly persons as compared to young, healthy, physically active young adults (Roubenoff, 2001). This reduction in muscle mass is known as sarcopenia (from the Greek meaning poverty of flesh), and is distinct from muscle loss due to disease or starvation. One population-based study estimated that the prevalence of sarcopenia rises from 13–24% in individuals under the age of 70 years to greater than 50% in persons over the age of 80 years (Baumgartner et al., 1998). Sarcopenia is of great consequence to older persons because it is associated with tremendous increases in functional disability and frailty. Older sarcopenic men are reported to have 4.1 times higher rates and women 3.6 times higher rates of disability than their gender-specific counterparts with normal muscle mass (Baumgartner et al., 1998).

The total cross-sectional area of skeletal muscle is reported to decrease by as much as 40% between the ages of 20 and 60 years (Doherty, 2003), with the greatest loss occurring in the lower limbs (Doherty, 2003; Vandervoot & Symons, 2001). Men are known to have greater total muscle mass than women; however, men experience greater relative muscle loss with age than do their female counterparts (Janssen, Heymsfield, Wang, & Ross, 2000). The reason for this gender difference has not been clearly defined, but it is postulated to relate to hormonal factors (Janssen et al., 2000). Although men experience greater relative muscle loss, it has been noted that sarcopenia may be of greater concern for older women given their longer life expectancy and higher rates of disability in old age (Roubenoff & Hughes, 2000). Gender is not the only factor contributing to differences in the rate of sarcopenia. The loss of muscle mass is highly individualized and greatly dependent upon genetic, lifestyle, and other factors that influence the varied mechanisms proposed to underlie sarcopenia. The most commonly proposed mechanisms include a decline in the number and size of muscle fibers, loss of motor units (described below), hormonal influences, altered protein synthesis, nutritional factors, and lack of physical activity.

Changes in Muscle Fibers

With age, there is an overall loss in the number of both fast- and slow-twitch muscle fibers. By the ninth decade, approximately 50% fewer muscle fibers are present in the vastus lateralis muscle (the lateral portion of the quadriceps) than are observed in the same muscle of a 20-year-old (Lexell, Taylor, & Sjostrom, 1988). In addition, a reduction in the size of muscle fibers has been observed, with the greatest reduction seen in fast-twitch muscle fibers. Reduction in the size of fast-twitch fibers ranges from 20% to 50% with age, whereas slow-twitch fibers have been shown to reduce in size by only 1% to 25% as a person ages (Doherty, 2003).

Loss of Motor Units

Muscle fibers are innervated by motor nerves, which extend from the spinal cord. Each nerve innervates several muscle fibers. The combination of a single nerve and all the fibers it innervates is known as a motor unit, and it is this motor unit that allows muscles to contract. Beginning about the seventh decade of an individual's life, the number of functional motor units begins to decline precipitously (Vandervoot & Symons, 2001). One group of researchers found that the estimated number of motor units in the bicep-brachialis muscle declined by nearly half, from an average of 911 motor units in subjects less than 60 years of age to 479 in subjects older than 60 years of age (Brown, Strong, & Snow, 1988). A similar degree of motor unit loss was shown in a group of subjects ages 60 to 80 years compared with a group of subjects ages 20 to 40 years (Doherty & Brown, 1993).

The loss of motor units with age is due to an age-related loss of muscle innervation (Deschenes, 2004). As motor units are lost, surviving motor nerves adopt muscle fibers that have been abandoned due to their loss of innervation (Roubenoff, 2001). This results in an increase in the size of the adopting motor unit. Thus, older persons generally have larger, yet less efficient, motor units than do younger persons (Roubenoff, 2001). Because these enlarged motor units are now responsible for the contraction of a greater number of muscles, they are generally less efficient. This inefficiency can lead to tremors and weakness (Enoka, 1997) and, together with the atrophy of fast-twitch muscle fibers, can result in a decline in coordinated muscle action (Morley, Baumgartner, Roubenoff, Mayer, & Nair, 2001). Furthermore, abandoned muscle fibers that are not adopted by surviving motor units begin to atrophy as a result of disuse secondary to their loss of innervation. This atrophy contributes to an overall loss of muscle mass. Muscle atrophy secondary to nerve cell death is clearly demonstrated through the loss of muscle mass observed in persons who have suffered a stroke (Roubenoff, 2001).

Hormonal Influences

Estrogen and testosterone are anabolic hormones—hormones that promote the build-up of muscle. With age, levels of these hormones decline, thereby contributing to muscle atrophy and sarcopenia. Accelerated loss of muscle around the time of menopause lends support to the idea that estrogen may play a role in the maintenance of muscle mass (Poehlman, Toth, & Gardner, 1995). There is evidence supporting estrogen replacement therapy as a means of attenuating the loss of muscle mass among older women (Dionne, Kinaman, & Poehlman, 2000; Phillips, Rook, Siddle, Bruce, & Woledge,1993). However, some research suggests that the beneficial effects of estrogen replacement are most pronounced in the perimenopausal period and may have little to no effect on the loss of muscle mass among postmenopausal women (Doherty, 2003). Among older men, testosterone supplementation has been shown to increase muscle mass; however, studies performed to date have been conducted among healthy older men. It is not known whether testosterone supplementation would have the same beneficial effects on muscle mass in older men with physical impairments, chronic disease, or frailty (Bhasin, 2003). Testosterone has also been shown to increase muscle strength among elderly women (Davis, McCloud, Strauss, & Burger, 1995).

Growth hormone (GH) (see "The Endocrine System" earlier in this chapter) is another anabolic hormone that declines with age. The decline in GH begins during the fourth decade of life and parallels the decline in muscle mass (Roubenoff, 2001). Because of the strong association between GH and muscle mass, administration of GH has been suggested as a potential method by which age-related loss of muscle mass might be attenuated. However, research investigating the effects of GH on muscle mass has produced equivocal results, and there is no evidence that GH administration results in any increase in muscle strength (Borst, 2004). In addition, the use of GH is accompanied by numerous side effects including fluid retention, hypotension, and carpal tunnel syndrome, and these side effects are reported to be more severe among older persons (Borst, 2004). Given the equivocal results regarding its efficacy as well as the side effects associated with its use, GH is not recommended as an intervention for sarcopenia (Doherty, 2003).

Protein Synthesis

After exclusion of water, protein is the primary component of skeletal muscle and accounts for approximately 20% of its weight (Proctor, Balagopal, & Nair, 1998). Furthermore, muscle is the body's largest repository for protein (Balagopal et al., 1997; Proctor et al., 1998). When protein breakdown within the body exceeds protein synthesis, muscle atrophy occurs. Some research findings suggest that aging is associated with a reduced capacity of skeletal muscle to synthesize protein. Such a reduction is likely to lead to a decrease in muscle mass among elderly persons. However, other research (Volpi, Sheffield-Moore, Rasmussen, & Wolfe, 2001) has found no difference in the synthesis rate of muscle protein with age. Thus, further studies are needed to elucidate the role that protein synthesis plays in sarcopenia.

Nutritional Factors

Food intake declines with age, with greater decline occurring among men than women (Morley et al., 2001). This decline is often referred to as the anorexia of aging, and is hypothesized to be associated with a decrease in the senses of smell and taste as well as an earlier rate of satiation with age (Morley et al., 2001). It is thought that the anorexia of aging may result in protein intake below the level necessary to maintain muscle mass and consequently contribute to sarcopenia (Morley et al., 2001). However, the degree to which alterations in protein intake with age may play a role in age-related loss of muscle mass is unknown and requires further study.

Muscle Strength

Loss of muscle strength, the muscle's capacity to generate force, is thought to be secondary to declines in muscle mass (Ivey et al., 2000), and decreases in muscle strength are seen with advancing age. Data from one study demonstrated that 71% of men between the ages of 40 and 59 and 85% of men age 60 or older had declines in muscle strength over a 9-year period (Kallman, Plato, & Tobin, 1990). Age-related decreases in strength are reported to range from 20–40%, with even greater decreases of 50% or more occurring in persons in their ninth decade or beyond (Doherty, 2003). Older men experience greater absolute declines in muscle strength than women; however, because men have greater total muscle mass than women, relative losses in strength are similar between males and females (Doherty, 2003). The rate at which the decline in muscle strength occurs has not been well defined, but longitudinal studies have shown rates of strength loss of about 1–3% per year (Doherty, 2003).

Muscle Quality

In addition to declines in muscle mass and strength, advancing age is also associated with a loss of muscle quality, strength generated per unit of muscle mass. However, research shows that age-related declines in muscle quality differ by both gender and muscle group. A study (Lynch et al., 1999) of arm and leg muscle quality in men and women found that age-related differences in arm muscle quality declined more among males than females, yet leg muscle quality declined at similar rates among both genders. In addition, among men the rates of decline of leg and arm muscle quality were similar. However, among women there was a greater rate of decline of leg muscle quality than arm muscle quality. Thus, age-related decline in muscle quality is highly variable, and studies examining this decline should be vigilant to include various muscle groups as well as subjects of both genders.

Resistance Training and Aging Muscle

Older persons who are less physically active have less muscle mass and greater rates of disability than persons who remain physically active as they age (Evans, 2002). There is a large body of evidence demonstrating that exercise cannot only slow or prevent muscle loss with age, but also increase muscle mass as well as muscle strength among older persons. Resistance exercise, exercise aimed at increasing the force generated by muscle, has been shown to have the most beneficial effects on aging muscle. One study (Frontera, Meredith, O'Reilly, Knuttgen, & Evans, 1988) of 66-year-old men found that a 12-week program of resistance training resulted in significant increases in the cross-sectional area of both fast-twitch and slow-twitch muscle fibers. In addition, muscle strength improved significantly. Even among very elderly persons, resistance exercise has shown benefits for age-related changes in muscle. An 8-week resistance training program conducted among men and women in their 90s resulted in a 15% increase in muscle cross-sectional area and a nearly 175% increase in the amount of weight subjects were capable of lifting (Fiatarone et al., 1990). Numerous other studies have shown that resistance training programs of 10 to 12 weeks duration, with training 2–3 days per week, result in significant increases in muscle strength among older persons (Doherty, 2003). It has been reported that resistance training may restore approximately 75% of lost muscle mass and 40% of lost muscle strength (Roubenoff, 2003).

Resistance training has also been shown to improve muscle quality. Following a 9-week training program, older men and women showed statistically significant increases in muscle quality. Furthermore, subsequent to the initial 9-week program there was a 31-week detraining period after which levels of muscle quality remained significantly greater than levels measured before the start of the 9-week program (Ivey et al., 2000).

Finally, there is also evidence to support an increase in protein synthesis with resistance exercise. One study reported an approximately 50% increase in protein synthesis among 65- to 75-year-old men following a 16-week progressive resistance training program (Yarasheski, Zackwieja, Campbell, & Bier, 1995). Improvements in protein synthesis have also been demonstrated among frail elderly men and women ages 76–92 years (Yarasheski et al., 1999). Other research has reported increases in protein synthesis of over 100% following resistance training (Hasten, Pak-Loduca, Obert, & Yarasheski, 2000).

The plethora of benefits to muscle that result from resistance training demonstrate the extreme importance of regular physical activity, especially of the resistance type, among aging men and women. It is no wonder that many have cited resistance training as the most important factor in preventing and even reversing the losses in muscle mass, strength, and power that come with advancing age.

APPENDIX 7-B

The Cornell Note-Taking System: Step-Wise Approach

As with most other tasks in nursing school and nursing, you want to approach note taking systematically. The Cornell note-taking system is one of the most commonly used systems and is fairly easy to learn. In this section a brief discussion of the Cornell note-taking system is provided.

Before the Lecture
Part of using the Cornell system involves preparation. The first step in your preparation involves getting rid of your spiral notebook and getting yourself a three-ring binder and loose-leaf notebook paper. If you do not want to purchase loose-leaf notebook paper, you can use plain white paper, but you will need a three-hole punch because you will need to be able to keep all of your notes in the same binder. You will only be using one side of the paper to take notes.

In preparation for note taking, use a ruler to draw a line down the left side of your paper (see Figure 7-1). This line should be between 2 and 3 inches from the left edge of the sheet. As you will see, the notes you take in class will be taken on the right side of the line, and the left side is what is known as the *recall column*. In this column you will put key words and phrases.

Figure 7-1   Lecture Notes in the Cornell System

2½"	6"
physical growth and development of 4–6 month old	4–6 months: around 4 months growth rate slows to approx. 20g/day primitive reflexes start to diminish–red flag if primitive reflexes do not no head lag when pulled to sitting; sits with support vision–follow an object to a full arc of 180 degrees purposeful movements emerge → improved fine motor • Hold objects • Intentional rolling • ↑ Head control • feeds self (bottle)
personal-social development of 6–8 month old What is pincer grasp? What is palmar grasp?	6-8 months: personal-social • stranger anxiety fine motor: • crude pincer grasp **know pincer grasp–infant reaches for an object using the thumb and forefinger palmar grasp–infant reaches for an object using the palm of the hand, rakes object in with fingertips

During the Lecture

You are now ready to start taking notes. The format of the notes that you put in the right column may consist of short phrases and definitions, short sentences, or brief paragraphs. With the Cornell system the types of notes you take depends on the structure and content of the material that is being presented in lecture. You will figure out what format works best for each of your classes with time. For example, when taking notes in your microbiology course, you might use short phrases and definitions; and when taking notes in your pediatric theory course, you might use topics and paragraphs. What is most important is that (1) you focus on writing telegraphic sentences or a streamlined version of the main points of the lecture by leaving out unnecessary words (e.g., *a*, *the*, and unimportant verbs) and using only key words, and (2) your notes are clear enough and complete enough that they will make sense to you several weeks after taking them. To achieve these goals you need to keep your focus on the main ideas, use abbreviations, leave plenty of space, and write legibly.

After the Lecture

Ideally you will make time to read through your notes right after class; however, that is not always possible, so make it a priority to go over your notes before the end of the day. After reading your notes, clean up areas that need attention such as illegible scribbles or details that you left blank. Finally, highlight the words that contain the main ideas, terms, or concepts that you want to remember.

After this step you are ready to make use of the recall column of your notes. In this column you write down the key words and phrases that connect the facts and ideas that you gained from your lecture with how you recall these facts and ideas upon reflection. Reflect on each of the topics or short paragraphs in your notes, and come up with a few words that capture what was presented in class. Essentially, what you write in the recall column is a condensed summation of the notes you took during the lecture. What is most important about the condensed summation is that you think about the points that were made in class, and you summarize the point in your own words.

Recitation, Reflection, and Recapitulation

After you have written your condensed summation in the recall column, you begin the process of moving the information you received during the lecture from your short-term memory into your long-term memory. You accomplish this transfer by taking the time to recite your notes aloud. Cover up the right side of your sheet—where your notes are—with a blank piece of paper; for each of the condensed summations in your recall column, recite aloud all of the concepts and ideas that you can from the lecture. As you speak, think about what you are saying and what it means. Uncover the right side of the sheet and check what you said with what is written on the right side. In your review think about the relevance of the information. Ask yourself such questions as: How does this information fit with what I already know from my previous lectures, reading, or clinical experience? How can I apply what I have learned in my nursing care? Finally, on the last page of your notes write a summary of the lecture that summarizes the main points you want to remember. This is not a rewrite of your notes. You are using your own words to summarize the key points that help with remembering the material and provide a very useful study guide.

Following the steps of the Cornell system can help you with retaining the information from your lectures; however, to consolidate this information in your memory you need to allocate several minutes each day to review your notes. During these review sessions you need to follow the steps of recitation and reflection discussed above.

EIGHT

Participating in an Online Course

The number of college students taking online courses continues to rise. A recent report found that more than 3 million college students in the United States were taking at least one online course during the fall 2005 term, which is a substantial increase over the 2.3 million reported the previous year (Allen & Seaman, 2006). I teach at least one Web-based course each semester, and all of the classroom-based courses I teach at Rutgers University have some Web-based materials (e.g., lectures, reading assignments). You may never take a Web-based or Web-enhanced course as a nursing student; however, because of the growing number of students taking Web-based and Web-enhanced courses and my own experiences teaching these types of courses, I think it is worthwhile to provide some background on online courses and some recommendations on how to make the most of this learning experience.

Advantages of Online Courses

There are several advantages associated with online courses for students. For example, in most cases, as long as you have a computer and an Internet connection, you can participate in an online course without being on campus or even in the same country. This is particularly relevant for students who do not live on campus and would have to spend time and money traveling to classes. Another advantage of most online courses is that they are *asynchronous* (there are no fixed meeting times), which allows students to participate in the course at a time that fits within their schedule. Finally, the structure of most online courses requires regular and consistent participation in online discussions and the submission of weekly assignments that force students to stay engaged with the course content.

Disadvantages of Online Courses

Although there are distinct advantages to online learning, students do have to make adjustments in their approach to learning, which can be challenging. For example, many students report feeling isolated and have to find new ways to connect with their online classmates and faculty such as phone calls, e-mails, and synchronous chat rooms. In addition, for some students the flexibility of online learning can make it easier to procrastinate and fall behind on assignments. Finally, some students have a difficult time adjusting to the technology used in online classes such as e-mail, electronic drop boxes, and document sharing.

Recommendations

Following the recommendations discussed below will help you avoid some of the biggest pitfalls of online courses.

Take the Tutorial

There are a number of Web-based software systems (e.g., Blackboard, eCollege) through which online content can be offered. Each of the systems has a great deal in common in terms of how they function; however, technical requirements, accessing the course content, and performing tasks such as e-mailing a professor or participating in an online chat are slightly different within each software system. Consequently, taking the time to familiarize yourself with the particular system that you are using may save time in the long run.

Make Sure You Check Your E-Mail

Web-based courses require the free flow of e-mail between students and the faculty teaching the course. Many students have personal e-mail accounts that they prefer to use rather than the institutional accounts they were assigned through their nursing school. When students are registered in the course, most of the Web-based software systems use the institutional e-mail account as the default e-mail account. This becomes a problem when your professor sends an e-mail to all those enrolled in the online course, and you do not receive it because you only check e-mail delivered to your personal account and do not check your assigned institutional account. On some of the Web-based software systems, you can change your e-mail address from your institutional e-mail address to your personal account. If changing your default e-mail is not possible and you are not confident in your ability to reliably check your institutional account, many e-mail systems have features that allow you to forward your e-mail to another account. This would allow you to have all your e-mail from your assigned institutional account forwarded to your personal e-mail account. Whatever the case, be proactive: do not wait until several weeks into the semester to determine that you are not receiving class-related e-mails.

Understand What the Expectations Are for Your Class

In contrast to traditional classroom-based courses, online courses usually involve weekly (and sometimes bi-weekly) assignments. These assignments may include Web-based journal entries, short writing assignments, and contributions to discussion boards.

Sidebar 8-1

Take The Tutorial

If there is an online tutorial for a course, take the tutorial. Find out the platform that will be used for the course, such as Blackboard. Make sure that you know how to use Blackboard *before* you take the course; otherwise, you will waste precious time that you will need to do your assignments. Keep to the schedule established by the professor for discussion postings, presentations, and assignments. It is particularly important for younger students to take these tutorials. Many younger students feel that because they have been using computers to play games, surf the Internet, and send e-mail that they know everything about computers, and consequently they do not take the online tutorial. This is a mistake. Students should take the online tutorial for the different online software platforms (e.g., Blackboard, eCollege) and learn how these systems operate.

Jeanne Ruggiero, PhD, RN, APN-C
Assistant Professor,
College of Nursing
Seton Hall University

You need to determine from the first day of the course what these assignments are and how they are submitted. For example, some professors prefer to have you submit your assignments electronically in the course "drop box," while others prefer to have the assignment sent as an e-mail attachment. In addition to weekly course assignments, you may have exams. Some professors may require that you travel to campus to take the exam, while others will offer the exams online. Finally, some faculty teaching online courses require that students participate in synchronous chats throughout the semester, which means that you will have to be in front of a computer at that time to participate.

Develop an Online Social Network with Faculty and Classmates

As discussed, adjusting to not seeing the faces and hearing the voices of classmates and faculty can make one feel isolated in the online learning environment. Simply because the majority of content in a course is delivered online does not mean that students cannot initiate contacts in the real world. For example, if you feel isolated or would like more contact with fellow classmates, there is a good chance that other students in the class share that feeling. There is nothing wrong with sending an e-mail to fellow classmates and inquiring whether they would like to meet on campus or at a mutually convenient spot to talk about the class, work on a project, or study for an exam. Students interested in more interpersonal contact can also ask online professors if office hours on campus are available or if they can arrange a time to discuss course concepts during a telephone conference.

Contribute to the Learning Environment

In addition to the assignments and exams, another important component of most on-line courses are asynchronous threaded discussions and synchronous chats. These discussions provide an important platform for you to learn by sharing ideas with other students in the class, and they provide your professor with an opportunity to evaluate what you are learning. When you are deciding what to post in these threaded discussions, ask yourself, "Am I adding any new information?" The value of your comments (and how they are evaluated by your professor) is the extent to which they broaden or deepen understanding. If you are posting information that has already been covered, then you are not expanding or enhancing the discussion. The same goes for posting such comments as, "I agree with what has been said."

Real-World Snapshot 8-1

Be Constructive in Online Threaded Discussions

A student enrolled in an online course that I taught really turned me off because she was unnecessarily critical and harsh toward other students. For example, she posted responses to other students like, "Your response was ridiculous," and "I think you need to read the book." She just made the online environment nonconducive to learning. Students are graded on the extent to which they contribute to a productive learning environment, and comments like those posted by this student detract from such.

Cynthia Ayres, PhD, RN
Assistant Professor, College of Nursing
Rutgers, The State University of New Jersey

Online discussions and chats can provide great opportunities for learning. Think of online discussions as a tree. The trunk of the tree is where the discussion begins. In some online nursing courses that I have taught, I have provided a case study and a few questions as the starting point for the discussion. Usually, the first couple of posts will answer the case study questions and compose the trunk of the tree. After the initial questions have been sorted out, new questions emerge and become branches of the tree. For example, if the central topic is common pediatric dermatological conditions and the cases have been covered sufficiently, one might consider discussing other related topics such as tinea (versicolor, cruris, capitis), the treatment options for tinea, the treatment options for other skin conditions, and so on.

Real-World Snapshot 8-2

Don't Be a Last Minute Online "Poster"

Don't wait until the last day to post a response in online discussions. I take points off for that because students who wait until the last day are not contributing to the learning environment, and often they are just rehashing posts that have been made earlier in the discussion.

Cynthia Ayres, PhD, RN
Assistant Professor, College of Nursing
Rutgers, The State University of New Jersey

Below is an example of a good exchange between students in an online discussion. As you can see, a post does not need to be lengthy to be of value. What makes these posts valuable to the learning process is that the students reference studies, they take the discussion in new directions, and they summarize the information and apply it to practice.

Sample Online Discussion

Student A:

I found this article and thought it would be of interest for this unit discussion. The authors sought to answer the question: In patients with fungal infections of the skin of the foot (tinea pedis), does oral treatment eradicate the infection? Studies were identified through a literature search of several databases. 12 trials were included and evaluated 5 antifungal treatments. Their results showed that in patients with fungal infections of the skin of the foot, terbinafine or itraconazole eradicate infection better than placebo, and terbinafine is better than griseofulvin. Different azoles and different doses of fluconazole did not differ in effectiveness.[1]

Student B:

I read an interesting study that reviewed the occurrence of loss of taste by patients being tested with Terbinafine for fungal infection. The study albeit small and the first published (as per the authors) confirmed loss in all four major taste qualities and further suggested that olfactory dysfunction was not involved. Further research was encouraged by the authors.[2]

---

1. Harkless, G. E. (2002). Review: Oral antifungal drugs promote cure of fungal infections of the foot. *Evidence-Based Nursing, 5*(4), 108.
2. Doty, R., & Haxel, B. (2005). Objective assessment of Terbinafine induced taste loss. *Laryngoscope, 115*, 2035–2037.

The importance of summarizing the evidence that one includes in threaded discussions and applying it to practice cannot be overstated. Many students participating in online courses find useful information; however, rather than summarizing the information for their classmates, they cut and paste large chunks of the research study into the threaded discussion or they include only the reference to the study. Threaded discussions are like potluck meals where all the guests bring some dish that they have prepared for everyone else to eat, and cutting and pasting large chunks of information or providing only the references to articles is like bringing a frozen chicken or an uncooked pie to one of these meals. Don't be one of those guests in threaded discussions; add something to the discussion that your classmates can benefit from immediately.

Reference

Allen, E. A., & Seaman, J. (2006). *Making the grade: Online education in the United States, 2006.* Retrieved July 26, 2007, from http://www.sloan-c.org/publications/survey/pdf/making_the_grade.pdf

NINE

How to Make a Presentation in Nursing School

Nursing programs differ in how many opportunities are provided for students to make oral presentations; however, it is virtually guaranteed that at some point during your nursing education you are going to have to make a presentation. This section provides some basic tips for developing and delivering presentations.

Preparing a Presentation

In nursing school, you will often be required to present a case study on a patient or a summary of a paper that you are submitting in the class. If and when you go to graduate school, these in-class presentations can be lengthy, but in nursing school your time will probably be limited (10–15 minutes). A growing number of classrooms are equipped with LCD projectors and computers loaded with Microsoft PowerPoint, and you will probably be given the option to present your material using these tools. While many speakers spend too much time doing impressive things with PowerPoint (music, graphics, etc.) and too little time saying something valuable,

PowerPoint can be useful in organizing and presenting a talk.[1] This discussion assumes you will be using PowerPoint, even if you will only be using it to organize your talk.

Tell a Story

There are a few simple guidelines that will help you in crafting your presentation. First, you should think of your presentation as a story. Like every good story, yours will have a beginning, middle, and end. In the beginning of your story inform the audience what you are going to do, in the middle of the story you should do what you told the audience you would do, and at the end of the story you tell the audience what you just did. It may sound like a simple formula—and it is—but if you apply the formula thoughtfully the results can be impressive.

Rule of Three

Another important point to keep in mind is to aim to make only two or three important points in a talk because it is easy to overwhelm or frustrate an audience with too much information or detail in an oral presentation. Unlike information that is presented in written form, in an oral presentation the listener has no control over the flow of information. In contrast, a reader has all the control. For example, readers can gloss over sections that are not interesting and focus on those sections that are of interest or return to a previous section if a detail was missed. One way that you can decrease the likelihood of your listener feeling overwhelmed is by limiting the amount of information that you present. Realistically, they are going to remember only a few points, so why not have them remember the information that you think is most important. For example, if you were preparing a talk on the reasons you want to become a nurse, you might choose to focus on your interest in science and health, your passion for working with people, and an early experience you had in the hospital.

So how do you drive these points home? Imagine you are given a two-part assignment in your pediatric theory course that involves writing a paper on a health problem during infancy and making a 10–15 minute oral presentation on this problem. You have chosen infantile colic, which is a term used to describe an infant who is healthy

---

[1]It is important to note that PowerPoint is not universally admired. In his book *Beautiful Evidence* (2006), Edward Tufte writes a thoughtful and disapproving critique of PowerPoint that highlights how this software has compromised the transmission of information.

and well fed but has excessive irritability, crying, or fussiness. You have already done your research and written a paper that defines what colic is, discusses the suspected causes of colic, and explains the nonpharmacologic and pharmacologic management of colic. Because you have done all of this work, the temptation is to present all of this information as part of your oral presentation. In fact, what students do frequently is to cut the information from their paper and paste it into a PowerPoint slide. The result is that, instead of making an oral presentation of their work, these students end up reading slide after slide until they have gone through their entire paper. The class and instructor politely clap afterwards. While this may get you a passing grade, you have not developed any skills in presenting information and, depending on your career choices in nursing, these skills may be very important. Moreover, you have wasted an opportunity to educate your audience (fellow students, instructor). After all, you spent a considerable amount of time reviewing the evidence regarding infantile colic; you do not know everything, but you know more than your classmates and probably your instructor on this topic, so why not share what you know?

What to Say

Begin preparing your presentation by figuring out what you want to say. You have only 10–15 minutes, and, as discussed, your goal is to hammer home a few key points. It is important to remember that although you want your audience to feel like you are speaking to them, retention is best when the talk proceeds slowly at about 100–125 words per minute (a conversation proceeds at about three times that rate). You need to choose two or three relevant conceptual issues from your paper to include in your discussion. Imagine the goals for your talk might be for your audience to understand: the normal patterns of crying during infancy, the major criteria used to define colic, and teaching for parents of an infant with colic. If your audience leaves your talk remembering these points, you will have been successful. Now that you have chosen the major points of your talk, you can begin the process of laying out your talk in PowerPoint and using the formula discussed above: tell them what you are going to say, say it, and tell them what you said.

Developing Your Talk

There is a great deal of information on the Internet discussing how to make the best use of PowerPoint. Radel and Massoth (1999) offer four pieces of advice for making effective visual presentations:

1. Make it big—Your presentation should look outrageously large on your computer screen. If it doesn't, it is too small. All of the headings should be 44 point font, and the text should be 32 point font.
2. Keep it simple—The audience should be able to absorb the text or graphic of your slide in about 5 seconds. To stick to this rule you have to limit the amount of information that you convey on each slide.
3. Make it clear—If the audience has to struggle to figure out what is on the slide, then they are not listening to what you have to say. Radel and Massoth offer a number of suggestions for slide layout, font size, color schemes, and the use of color for emphasis.
4. Be consistent—As Radel and Massoth advise, "Be consistent in thought, deed, and action." What does this mean? No curveballs for your audience; use the story format that was discussed earlier, and stick to it.

The next section follows a sample oral presentation slide by slide.

1

> # Infantile colic: A nursing approach
>
> Joe Bagofdonuts
> Pediatric Theory
> Nursing School

Slide 1 is the title slide, which includes the title of your presentation, your name, and the course in which you are delivering the presentation.

2

> ## Overview
>
> - Crying babies
>   - Anecdote/joke
>   - Why should we care as nurses?
> - Learning expectancies
>   - the normal patterns of crying during infancy
>   - the major criteria used to define colic
>   - teaching for parents of an infant with colic

Slide 2 is the overview. Right away you want to orient the audience as to what you expect them to get out of this presentation—tell them what you are going to do and what you want them to learn. Plan on using the slides as prompts to remind you what you are going to talk about and to give the audience an idea of what you are talking about. While many presenters cram everything they want to say onto the slide and then read the slide, resist this temptation. To be able to use the slides in this manner, you will have to practice the presentation several times (10 times through is a good goal) before presenting it to your intended audience.

Sidebar 9-1

Practicing Your Presentation

As with preparing for a test or learning to hit a tennis ball, there is little benefit to "cramming." You are going to do better on your calculus test if you spread your study sessions out over a couple of days instead of waiting until the day before the test. You are going to develop a better backhand in tennis by spending 30 minutes a day for four consecutive days than 2 hours in one day. The same principle is true of preparing to speak in public: a few short practice sessions prior to the event are better than a lengthy practice session the day before you have to present. Here are some other guidelines for practicing your speech:

- Do not just read your presentation to yourself. Your presentation is going to sound different in your head than it will when you speak it aloud to an audience; consequently, find an audience to deliver your talk. It is great if you practice your talk in front of someone who knows or cares about the topic of your presentation, but that is not as important as finding someone who will sit and listen. It can be a significant other, a friend, or a relative.
- Ask someone in your practice audience to critique the process elements of your speech. Feedback you want from your practice audience includes: How many minutes does my presentation take? How was my rate of speaking? Did I speak too fast or too slow? Were you able to understand everything that I said, or did I mumble at times? How was my eye contact? Did I look at my audience, or was I looking at the floor?
- After you start your talk, go all the way through it. Make a mental note of the areas you want to revise, but keep on going through the talk.

Before giving an overview for the talk, you might try to personalize the talk and let the audience know why this topic matters by saying something like the following:

In the next 10 minutes I will be talking about crying during infancy. Specifically, I will discuss infantile colic. My interest in this topic comes from my adventures in babysitting and how frustrating it was when I was unable to soothe a crying infant. In fact, I left the babysitting profession at the tender age of 14 after a couple of experiences with one particularly fussy baby named Jake. He would cry from the moment his parents left until they returned home. I couldn't take Jake.

My experiences with Jake have given me empathy for parents of extremely fussy babies. The sound of a crying baby is meant to get the attention of adults, and I am sure it wears on adults. In fact there is some evidence to suggest that extremely fussy babies are more likely to be abused than less fussy babies. Consequently, as nurses, it is important to be able to provide teaching to parents of infants who may be fussy.

3

> ### What are the normal patterns of crying during infancy?

Slide 3 (What are the normal patterns of crying during infancy?) is a title slide. Each of the three topics is introduced by a slide that orients the audience to what is to come next. I know that in Slide 2 I told the audience what was to be presented; however, consistency is important. This slide will stay on the screen for about 5 seconds.

4

> ## The normal crying patterns of a young infant
> - an average of 2.2 hours/ day
> - peaking at six weeks of age
> - gradually decreasing

Slide 4 (The normal crying patterns of a young infant) provides some basic information on the normal crying patterns of infants. As you see from the slide, only the key words are put on the slide.

5

What is infantile colic?

Slide 5 (What is infantile colic?) is another title slide introducing what is to follow.

6

How do you know it is infantile colic?

- A "diagnosis of exclusion"
- Baby is healthy
- Baby is well-fed

Slide 6 (How do you know it is infantile colic?) contains a question. I find that the talk becomes more conversational for me if I put questions on the slides. These questions serve as triggers, reminding me of what I want to discuss and making me feel like I am answering questions. In this slide it would be important to explain what is meant by a "diagnosis of exclusion." Don't be afraid to make the presentation more of a two-way street by tossing a question out to the audience. You might say, "Can anyone guess what is meant by a diagnosis of exclusion?" This keeps the audience on their toes and takes some of the pressure off you.

7

How do you know it is infantile colic?

The Rule of 3
- crying more than **3** hours a day
- at least **3** days a week
- for at least **3** weeks in a row

Slide 7 (How do you know it is infantile colic?) introduces the audience to a simple way of assessing whether an infant can be considered to be "colicky"—the rule of three (crying more than 3 hours a day, at least 3 days a week, 3 weeks in a row).

8

> ## Possible causes of colic?
>
> • Multifactorial
>   - It may be the result of a baby's sensitive temperament
>   - Immature nervous system
>   - Dietary factors (e.g., high carbohydrate diet)

Slide 8 (Possible causes colic?) lists only a single cause of colic. An important goal for any talk—whether you are speaking to a room full of rocket scientists or a sixth grade health class—is to strike the right balance. You do not want to overload the audience with too much information, but you want them to leave the presentation feeling like their time was well spent. There are other suspected causes of colic besides the ones mentioned in the slide; however, the goal of this talk is not to discuss every possible cause of colic. If the audience wants to know more about the different causes, they can look at the paper this talk is based on or do research on their own. It is often helpful to include a handout with references/bibliography.

9

> ## When is colic worst?
>
> • Late afternoon and evening
>   - occurs in prolonged bouts
>   - unpredictable and spontaneous

Slide 9 (When is colic worst?) presents an interesting piece of information regarding colic that nurses can include in their teaching to parents.

10

> ## Managing a "colicky" baby

Slide 10 (Managing a colicky baby) is another slide that lets your audience know that you are making a transition and switching gears from discussing colic to how to manage colic.

11

> # Soothing/behavioral management
> - Use a pacifier.
> - Gently rock the infant
> - Massage the infant's abdomen or back to help pass gas or stool
> - Play relaxing music or sing to the infant
> - Offer food
>   - Sometimes a colicky baby is just hungry.
> - Hold & cuddle the baby.
> - Try constant background sound or "white noise"

. Slide 11 (Soothing/behavioral management) lists one of the two principal approaches to managing infantile colic with nonpharmacologic strategies—soothing and behavioral changes. You might want to let your audience know that there are pharmacologic management options that you will not cover in this talk. Again, the audience can look at your paper or research pharmacologic management strategies independently.

12

> # Dietary/food changes
> - Changing formula
> - If breast-feeding, try eliminating certain foods from diet such as
>   - cow's milk, caffeinated drinks, and "gassy" foods
>   - broccoli, cauliflower, cabbage, beans

Slide 12 (Dietary/food changes) presents the second approach to managing infantile colic nonpharmacologically—making changes in the baby's diet, or if the baby is breast-fed, making changes in the mother's diet.

13

Dietary/food changes

- Try switching to a new type of bottle
  - a different nipple, a different shape, or a collapsible bag.

Slide 13 (Dietary/food changes) continues the topic with a related dietary change of changing the baby bottle.

14

Summary

- Average crying 2.2 hours a day
- Remember the Rule of 3
  - 3 hours a day, 3 days a week, 3 days in a row
- Behavioral and dietary changes to help parents manage
  - Feeding, soothing, eliminating gassy foods

Slide 14 (Summary) is a brief review of whatever you think is most important from the presentation. Many presenters neglect to include a summary slide, which leads to that awkward moment where the audience has to decide if you are done or if you lost your train of thought. Remember, you tell them what you are going to do, do it, and then tell them what you did.

An important thing to notice about this presentation is that it is pretty simple. While you have the option with PowerPoint to make text and images dance around the screen and to include audio and video, it is not necessary. In fact, it can be distracting. The audience may be waiting for the next round of graphical fireworks rather than focusing on the content of your talk. Moreover, to add the bells and whistles in PowerPoint requires a substantial amount of time. Your time would be better spent rehearsing your presentation. The importance of practicing what you plan to say cannot be overstated, and by practice I mean practice aloud in front of your significant other, parent, next-door neighbor, or roommate. If you rehearse the material and feel comfortable with it, you will do a much better job in presenting and you will not make the mistake of reading the slides.

Delivering a Presentation

Some people may have some personality qualities (e.g., extraversion, good sense of humor) or physical attributes (e.g., a pleasing vocal quality) that give them an advantage as a public speaker; however, as with other skills—shooting a basketball or playing the piano—no one is born knowing how to speak in public or give an oral presentation. The ability to speak in public improves with practice. Of course, the practice is meaningless if you have not prepared a presentation that is clear and informative. The previous section discussed how to prepare your presentations for nursing school and beyond. In this section you will learn how to improve your delivery of a presentation, including information on getting over your fears of speaking in public and connecting with your audience.

Real-World Snapshot 9-1

Top Five Reasons Not to Imagine
Your Audience in Their Underwear

5. This advice was made famous on the Brady Bunch television show, and you do not want to get your advice from the Brady Bunch family.
4. Not everyone wears underwear.
3. Your audience may not look good in their underwear, which would be a distraction.
2. Your audience may look good in their underwear, which would be a distraction.
1. You need to focus on sharing your story and connecting with your audience, not on underwear.

The Fear Factor

If you are like most people, you have some anxiety about speaking in public. A number of surveys show that adults in the United States are more fearful of speaking in public than death (Motley, 1988; Richmond & McCroskey, 1995). So when people say, "I would rather die than speak in public," there is a good chance that they are not exaggerating. In fact, many who report being fearful of public speaking experience physiological reactions that are similar to the reactions they would experience if they were in a life-or-death situation: heart rate acceleration, dry mouth, and increased bowel activity.

Why are we so afraid of public speaking? Research suggests that it has to do with a number of related factors. These factors all revolve around the fact that when we engage in the act of public speaking, we are in a situation in which we are being evaluated by others. We are self-conscious, and on some level we may not feel that what we have to say or how we express ourselves will be up to the expectations of our audience (Ayres, 1986). In addition, in contrast to most interpersonal communication, there is a *one-wayness* to public speaking situations in that all of the verbal communication flows from the speaker (Ayres, 1986). Finally, many people dread being the center of attention (Daly, Vangelisti, & Lawrence, 1989).

It is important to realize that the symptoms (e.g., sweating, rapid pulse, dry mouth, racing thoughts) of anxiety or nervousness that you feel before speaking publicly are entirely normal and felt to some degree by almost everyone prior to public speaking. These effects are related to the mass activation of the sympathetic system that releases adrenaline and prepares your body to deal with a threat. The obvious benefit of this response is that it provides you with a physical and mental charge that prepares you to take action. This is often termed the *fight-or-flight* response. Of course, your body does not know that the threat you face as a public speaker is not an animal that wants to make a meal of you or an enemy with a club but an audience who you worry will think less of you after hearing you speak. Keeping this in mind, what can you do to get beyond your performance anxiety and deliver a successful oral presentation?

Preparation and Practice

I have made the mistake of trying to deliver presentations as a student, as a professor, and as a scholar for which I did not practice adequately. At the end of these presentations, I have always felt a sense of regret. I regretted that I stressed myself out more than I had to because I did not practice my talk. In addition, I regretted that I wasted the time of my audience by not giving them something useful with the time that they gave me. Not practicing the presentation that you have gone to the effort of preparing is like preparing a gourmet meal and then deciding to serve it on paper plates rather than using your best table settings. As they say in the culinary world: presentation is everything. When you have practiced your presentation, you are much more able to get out of your own head and focus on the material that you are trying to deliver.

Get Yourself into the Flow

At some point in your life you have probably been engaged in some activity requiring skill—engaging in a sports contest, solving a puzzle, creating music or art—where you were performing at your best without even thinking about it. The psychologist Mihaly Csikszentmihalyi (pronounced CHICK-sent-me-high-ee) defined this state of mind as *flow* or the mental state of operation in which the person is fully immersed in what he or she is doing, characterized by a feeling of energized focus, full involvement, and success in the process of the activity (Csikszentmihalyi, 1990). In his investigations of flow, Csikszentmihalyi used interviews and data from the social sciences to demonstrate that we become more successful (and fulfilled) when we achieve flow or become absorbed in whatever activity we are engaged in. To calm your anxiety and get yourself into the flow state in the days and hours before your talk, you need to visualize positive outcomes. Every time you feel yourself starting to get anxious about speaking, think about what it will look and feel like when you are standing in front of the room. Imagine yourself standing in front of the audience, speaking confidently and comfortably, making good eye contact with your audience, and going through your talk smoothly. Remind yourself that you are prepared. A few minutes before your talk do some deep breathing exercises: breathe in through your nose, send the breath deep into your belly and breathe out through your mouth. Focus on the rise and fall of your stomach.

It Is Not About You, But What You Have to Say

No matter the outcome of your talk—complete flop or a huge success—you need to remind yourself that it is just an oral presentation, and you will still be the same person you were before the talk. You will look the same, your friends and family will still love you, and the people that do not care for you will still not care for you. If you had something worthwhile to say in your talk, some of your audience will remember that you had something worthwhile to say, but they will probably not remember exactly what you said for very long. If you had nothing worthwhile to say or you could not get your points across, there is nothing to remember. Consequently, the worst-case scenario for your talk in nursing school is that you get a low mark from your professor for your talk and no one in your class remembers what you said.

You Are the Expert

Although your talk is not about you, do not forget that you are the expert on what you are going to say. You know more about the topic you have prepared yourself to speak about than your audience (and probably your professor). Your classmates and your classroom professor may have some passing familiarity with the topic of your oral presentation, but you know a great deal more. Remind yourself that you are not in the hot seat. Because you are the expert on your topic, you are in the driver's seat.

Be Your (Ideal) Self

One mistake I have made (and I have seen other students make) is trying to speak like I thought a good speaker should speak rather than just speaking like the best version of me. What do I mean by the best version of myself? We all have different versions of ourselves, and most of us select the version of ourselves that suits the occasion. Consequently, the version of yourself on a first date is probably not the same version of yourself on a last date, and the version of yourself that is out at a party on Saturday night is probably not the same version of yourself that goes to church on Sunday morning. Your ideal self for the oral presentation is the self that speaks simply. Don't stress yourself out trying to use vocabulary and phrases that do not come easily to you. Your ideal self for the oral presentation speaks clearly, so don't mumble or rush your thoughts. Your ideal self also speaks confidently—the way you might speak if you were sharing a story at dinner with people that you like and who like you and who want you to tell a good story—so make eye contact, breathe, and focus on telling your story. As discussed in this book, we (nurses and nursing students) have a unique perspective on health and health care because of our educational background and our experiences in caring for patients and their families; consequently, it is important that we are prepared to share our stories.

References

Ayres, J. (1986). Perceptions of speaking ability: An explanation for stage fright. *Communication Education, 35,* 275–289.

Csikszentmihalyi, M. (1990). *Flow: The psychology of optimal experience.* New York: Harper & Row.

Daly, J. A., Vangelisti, A. L., & Lawrence, S. G. (1989). Self-focused attention and public speaking anxiety. *Personality and Individual Differences, 10,* 903–913.

Motley, M. T. (1988). Taking the terror out of talk: Thinking in terms of communication rather than performance helps us calm our biggest fear. *Psychology Today, 22*(1), 46–49.

Radel, J., & Massoth, C. (1999). *Designing effective visuals.* Retrieved April 7, 2007, from http://www.kumc.edu/SAH/OTEd/jradel/Effective_visuals/VisStrt.html

Richmond, V. P., & McCroskey, J. C. (1995). *Communication: Apprehension, avoidance, and effectiveness* (4th ed.). Scottsdale, AZ: Gorsuch Scarisbrick.

TEN

How to Write a Paper in Nursing School

As evidenced by the success of the television show *American Idol*, there are a great number of people who believe that they have a talent for singing. My wife loves the show so I have watched more than a few episodes. One characteristic of the contestants that I find interesting is that they all have a great deal of confidence in their singing abilities despite the fact that they report that they have had no formal training in singing and they do not practice singing. Most of the contestants think that they can sing, and they seem genuinely deflated when the judges review them poorly.

As a professor I work with students who possess the same kind of confidence about their writing. Most students think that they write well. I can relate to these students because not too many years ago I was one of those students. Despite the fact that very few papers that I wrote as an undergraduate, graduate, and doctoral student received great reviews, I felt that it was a shortcoming of the reviewer, and it was only a matter of time before my paper would be read by someone who could appreciate my gift as a thinker and see the beauty of my prose.

It was not until I started writing scientific papers for publication that I slowly became aware that writing was a skill like playing the piano or learning a foreign language: one improves with practice. As I struggled to improve my writing (I still struggle), I recall a remark made by a mentor of mine, "Writing is not a sign of intelligence. There are a lot of very smart people who write poorly." That comment was one of those "Eureka!" or epiphanal moments, and I only wish someone had told me that earlier. Had I believed that good writing requires constant effort to develop, I may have worked at expressing my thoughts more clearly rather than hoping that the reader could intuit what I intended to convey. What is important to know is that with practice and attention to a few basic guidelines you can improve your writing. Provided in this chapter are some tips on how to do so.

Writing in Nursing School

The topics in the papers that you will write as a nursing school student will be different from the papers you would write if you were getting a degree in political science or English literature. For example, as a nursing student, you might be required to write a paper on the ethical and legal aspects of do-not-resuscitate orders or how you would teach a 12-year-old newly diagnosed with diabetes to administer insulin. Despite these differences, good writing is good writing. Before delving into the recommendations for writing your papers in nursing school, there are two important points that you should keep in mind about these papers.

Most Professors Do Not Enjoy Grading Papers

First, I know this may come as a shock, but most educators do not look forward to reading students' papers. Your paper is an obstacle that is preventing your instructor from going to bed, working on research, going home, eating dinner, watching television, and so on. Your paper and the papers of your 30 or so classmates are in the way of this person's life because these papers have to be read and grades have to be assigned fairly. There may be some exceptions to this rule, but it is best to assume that the educator reading your paper would rather be doing something else (anything else).

You Are Dealing with a Nurse

Second, your professor in nursing school probably has a nursing education and a background working as a nurse. These experiences are called upon when reading your paper. What do I mean? Many nursing roles focus on being able to do quick and accurate assessments of patients. One skill that helps in this assessment is the ability to quickly identify abnormal findings or "red flags" in the human condition. Red flags are physiological and psychosocial findings that reflect poor health or an impending crisis such as nasal flaring and increased respirations in an infant or a 50-year-old man complaining of chest pain and jaw discomfort. In the world of nursing these red flags indicate the need for further evaluation and treatment. This skill of assessing red flags is readily transferable to the reading of papers, and it is likely that if someone with a nursing background is reading your paper, he or she is looking for red flags. In your paper these red flags indicate the need for the deduction of points from the final grade of your paper.

Where do these points come from? If your instructor is anything like me, he or she uses a scoring sheet for your paper. It might look something like Table 10-1.

Table 10-1   Grading Sheet: Evidence-Practice Paper

	Fall 200x
Name:	
Overall quality of writing (e.g., grammar, organization, sentence structure, proofreading):	• 25 points
Clinical question: • How did you refine your question?	• 15 points
Process of obtaining evidence: • What was your process? • How could it have been improved?	• 40 points
Critical appraisal of evidence • What did you find? • How will you use this evidence to guide your decisions?	• 20 points
Total	• 100 points

Scoring sheets allow your instructor to quickly assess the extent to which you followed the guidelines for the assignment. The scoring categories and number of points in each category are usually taken directly from the guidelines.

Preparing to Write Your Paper

Start with the Guidelines of the Paper

The course syllabus is your friend, and the guidelines for your paper will most likely be found on your syllabus. Find these guidelines and read them carefully. Your instructor has probably devoted some class time to discussing the paper, and you should integrate what was said in class with what is discussed in the syllabus. Take note of what questions you have been instructed to answer, when the paper is due, the maximum number of pages, and so on. One important point to remember about the suggested length of the paper: if your professor has instructed you to write a paper that should be "no more than x pages in length," you are shooting for 75–80% of that number. So if the guidelines say a maximum of 10 pages, your goal is to write a paper that is 7–8 pages because, as you will find, less is often more. This 75–80% rule usually gives you more than enough space to achieve the goals of the writing assignment if you are organized and economical in your writing, which is to your advantage because faculty members do not want to read papers that are padded with superfluous information.

Choose a Topic

In many of your nursing school classes, your professor will give you some idea of the range of topics. Look at these guidelines and find a topic that is (1) going to be of interest to you, and (2) makes you feel that you are going to learn something. The other point that you want to keep in mind at this stage of the process is that you do not have to love the topic of your paper. You are not writing a book or your dissertation. Do not get hung up on trying to find the perfect topic.

Focus Your Topic

If you are like most students, the topic that you have chosen is too broad and you are going to have to narrow it down. For example, imagine you have chosen respiratory syncytial virus (RSV)—which is the most common cause of viral lower respiratory tract infection in infants—as the topic for a paper you are writing in a pediatric theory course. Most of your papers in nursing school will be no more than 5–10 pages, so you will need to give some thought to exactly what you will discuss regarding RSV. Focus your topic according to what will help you the most when you are providing care for your patients. For the topic of RSV, this might include information on treatments to reduce the transmission of RSV or on how to teach families about what to expect in their child who has RSV. Think about your clinical experiences, discussions you had in class, or reading that you have done to focus your question. If you are having trouble, schedule a meeting with your professor as early in the semester as possible. During this discussion lay out your areas of interest and get feedback from your professor on what might be interesting to explore in a paper. Your professor will probably be able to steer you in a direction that connects with your interest, is focused, and is genuinely researchable.

Develop an Outline

Develop an outline of your paper using the guidelines of the assignment. Use the outline to structure the major headings for your paper. In most of your nursing school courses, your instructor wants to know how *you* are thinking and whether you can demonstrate through your writing that you are able to apply the major concepts of the course. So resist the temptation to start researching your topic until you have sketched out what you want to say and how it applies to the course. Many students who start researching before they have developed an outline end up with a paper that does not reflect their thinking because they have strung together articles and other publications in their paper as they try to account for all of the research that they have gathered. If you use your course notes and handouts to begin outlining your paper, you have a better chance of writing in a way that reflects your thoughts and keeps your paper tight and focused.

Researching Your Topic

Thanks to advances in technology, the research process becomes more convenient every year. Many students reading this book will have access to Internet sources that allow them to conduct their searches using a computer and make it unlikely that they will ever have to conduct manual searches for information in the library. Despite these advances, you still need a strategy for approaching the search process systematically.

Imagine you chose RSV in infants as your research topic. From your reading and class lectures you know that it is the leading cause of infant hospitalization, and premature babies or those with lung or heart problems have an especially high risk. For your paper you are required to develop a teaching plan for parents of infants hospitalized with RSV. You have sketched an outline of the topics that you want to cover in your teaching plan:

1. Basic pathophysiology
2. Clinical manifestations
3. Diagnosis
4. Clinical management
5. Prognosis

The outline above is pretty straightforward, and you could probably get all of the information that you need to write your paper from your textbook.

There are at least two good reasons that you should resist this temptation. First, your textbook is a *secondary source*, meaning it is a source that provides descriptions of studies prepared by someone other than the original researcher. The problem with secondary sources is that, as with most secondhand information, you are getting another's interpretation of primary information. Think of the telephone game that you may have played in which each successive participant secretly whispers to the next person a phrase or sentence whispered to him or her by the preceding participant. The message becomes progressively altered as each participant makes a small error in what is repeated. You want your information to be accurate; consequently, as a nursing student and nurse, your goal is to read *primary sources*. These are research reports written by the researcher who conducted the research.

In addition to providing you with information that is less likely to have been misinterpreted, another advantage of using primary sources over secondary sources such as your textbook is that your textbook contains some health information that was outdated even before it was published. Information in nursing and medicine changes quickly, and what was current when your textbook was published may have changed. By using primary sources you will be able to locate and reference the most current evidence.

The practice of using primary sources and the most current evidence to make decisions about patient care is referred to as *evidence-based practice (EBP)*. A thorough discussion of the history of the EBP movement, components of EBP, and relevance to nursing practice is beyond the scope of this book; however, Drs. Bernadette Melnyk and Ellen Fineout-Overholt (2005) wrote an excellent guide to EBP titled, *Evidence-Based Practice in Nursing and Healthcare: A Guide to Best Practice.* Most of the discussion below regarding EBP and conducting searches is based on this guide.

Searching for Information

As discussed above, the information in your textbook is secondhand and may be outdated. Consequently, in preparing papers during nursing school, your textbook should be used only to provide you with background information on your topic. What does that leave you with? You could go to the library and conduct your search for information via a print-based literature search; however, most students have access to Internet resources that make print-based literature searches and some manual searches unnecessary and an inefficient use of time.

Internet Search Engines

Searching for the information that you need through an Internet search engine such as Google or Yahoo is how many students begin their research process. Although this method of searching for information will provide you with a great number of sites mentioning your topic, most of these sites will include commercial products, information from advocacy groups, and other information that is designed for and by nonhealthcare professionals. Keep in mind that the Internet is an equal opportunity electronic bazaar, and anyone can put up a Web site with health information. While some of this information may be accurate and interesting, a substantial amount of this information is not. If you are reading this book, you are probably interested in developing a more sophisticated understanding of your health topic than would likely be provided on most of these types of Web sites. Moreover, sorting through these Web sites trying to separate the fact from the fiction is not the best use of your time. One exception to this general rule is Google Scholar, which can be a great resource if you know how to use the search engine to your advantage (see discussion below on searching).

Bibliographic Database

There are several other good Internet options to strategically and systematically search for information. One is to search bibliographic databases that contain short summaries, or abstracts, of publications and the author, title, and journal name. These bibliographic databases include the following:

- CINAHL—Contains references to material and studies relating to nursing, allied health, and medicine dating back to 1982

- MEDLINE—Similar to CINAHL, contains references to studies in medicine, nursing, and allied health
- PsycINFO—Contains references to studies and materials in psychology and related healthcare disciplines

Full-Text Databases
Depending on whether your institution has chosen to pay for a subscription to the online journal, you may be able to access full-text articles of the bibliographic databases mentioned above. These full-text databases offered through commercial vendors (e.g., Ovid, EbscoHost) include text, charts, graphs, and other illustrations.

Systematic Reviews
Another important source of reliable information are the systematic reviews found in the Cochrane Database of Systematic Reviews (CDSR) (www.cochrane.org) and the National Guideline Clearinghouse (NGC) (www.guidelines.gov). The CDSR contains systematic reviews, which are syntheses of studies that pertain to a common clinical question. The NGC contains systematically developed guidelines about a plan of care for a specific set of clinical circumstances (Melnyk & Fineout-Overholt, 2005). What makes these databases so valuable is that the studies and guidelines contained in these databases represent rigorous appraisal of numerous studies. Consequently, clinicians (and students) are able to find the best available clinical evidence in the shortest time. In essence, this is one-stop shopping. If you can find the information that you are looking for in this database, your search is over.

Guidelines for Searching
Most libraries and research textbooks have tutorials and extensive instructions on searching databases to locate information. This section provides a brief introduction on some of the basics of searching.

Start at the Top
As mentioned, if you can find the information that you are looking for in the CDSR or NGC, your search is over—so start there. Your institution may not have a subscription to the CDSR; try the NGC at www.guidelines.gov.

Search Terms
Most of the databases discussed allow you to use subject headings or keywords to search for information quickly. An example of subject headings includes those used by the National Library of Medicine for MEDLINE, which are referred to as MeSH

headings. MeSH headings can be found at the National Library of Medicine at www.nlm.nih.gov/pubs/factsheets/mesh.html. Each article in the database is associated with multiple MeSH headings and subheadings. Searching full-text databases using keywords (everyday words and expressions) can also lead to good results.

Boolean Searching

The terms *AND* and *OR* are known as Boolean operators and can be used to restrict or broaden a search. For example, if you were searching for information on RSV and entered the keyword RSV while using CINAHL software, your search would result in 252 hits. Entering the terms *RSV AND treatment* would narrow your results to 64 hits, and entering the terms *RSV AND treatment AND infants* would narrow your results to 33 hits. On the other hand if you entered the terms *RSV OR bronchiolitis,* you would expand your results to include 570 hits. I should note that these hits are for abstracts of the articles, not the full text. It is unlikely that you will be able to obtain every article for which you get a result.

Wildcard Characters

When searching the bibliographic databases using keywords, you can also improve your results by using *$* as part of the search term. For example, by using the *$* after the word *infant*, your search results would include all words that begin with infant such as infants and infantile.

Writing Your Paper

Start with the Core of the Paper

After choosing a topic, developing an outline, and gathering at least some of the research that you will need, it is time to start writing your paper. Do not make the mistake of taking a linear approach to writing your paper. For example, many students start the writing process by working on an introductory paragraph. This might feel like a reasonable place to start because it is the first section of your paper; however, you are more efficient by starting with the body of your paper for at least two reasons. First, by starting with the body of your paper, you are able to "hit the ground running" because the gathering of your research should have given you a pretty good idea of what the major themes are in your paper. Second, your ideas are going to evolve as you start writing, and by not starting with your introduction you save yourself the time you will have to spend rewriting your introduction.

Approach your paper like a crossword puzzle. In completing a crossword puzzle, there is no rule that you have to start with 1 Across, fill in those spaces, and move to 2 Across. You can complete the crossword puzzle in the way that works best for you. Employ the same strategy in your writing process. Use your outline to lay out the sections, and fill in those pieces that you have.

Keep Moving

Writing is a process, and initially your goal is to start getting your thoughts on the page. In the beginning of the process do not get bogged down with trying to find the right word or making sure that each sentence is perfectly coherent and grammatically correct. Keep the words and ideas flowing, and know that you will have to come back later to clean it up. Moreover, do not spend time on other activities that you can do later such as formatting references for American Psychological Association (APA) style or paraphrasing source material; these kinds of activities will block your flow. Instead, write notes to yourself as you move along like, "Put Smith quote here," that you can follow up on later. In addition, when you get stuck in a section, do not dwell; move on to a different section, and write a note to yourself like, "More here," or questions like, "What are the side effects?"

Do Not Neglect the Introductions and Conclusions

As with developing an oral presentation, when you write, tell your audience what you are going to do, do it, and tell them what you did. You want to make reading your paper as easy for your professor as possible, and telling the reader what you are going to do in the introduction and what you did in the conclusion makes it easy for your instructor to evaluate your paper. It does not matter if your paper is 2 pages or 50 pages; you want to give the reader some sense of what your goals are in the paper. For most of your papers the introduction can usually be accomplished in 1 or 2 sentences. For example:

> In this paper I will critique the research problem, review of literature, and conceptual framework discussed by Neu, Browne, and Vojir (2000) in their article, "The Impact of Two Transfer Techniques Used During Skin-to-Skin Care on the Physiologic and Behavioral Responses of Preterm Infants."

Telling the reader what you did in a concluding paragraph also improves your paper. As in the introduction, this can be done briefly:

Neu, Browne, and Vojir compared the effect of two different transfer methods on the physiologic stability of the infant. The goals of the study were clearly stated in the introduction and the authors' review of the literature was well organized and provided a rationale for the study. No conceptual framework was used in the study; however, the absence did not detract from the study's value.

As mentioned, the conclusion does not need to be lengthy; you are simply giving the reader a sense of closure. This can be done in a number of ways, such as summarizing how what you have written connects with your thesis or by discussing questions to be explored in future papers. What you do not want to do is leave the reader hanging by doing what many of us did in elementary school and writing "The End" or just stopping wherever your thoughts end.

Use Headings to Guide the Reader

Another way to improve the readability of your paper involves the use of headings to structure your paper. By using headings you are constantly orienting the reader as to what they should expect in the next section. In the care of children and families we call this "anticipatory guidance," and nurses provide anticipatory guidance to parents regarding the developmental milestones that are coming up "around the bend." This guidance involves information about changing patterns in sleep, diet, and elimination, and parents want this information because most people do not want surprises when it comes to parenting. The headings provide the same kind of guidance for the reader of your paper. The key to using the headings effectively is to use the paper guidelines to determine what headings you should use. If the guidelines required that you address the clinical implications, then include a heading "Clinical Implications."

Be Precise

Be selective in your word choice. Make sure the words you are using accurately reflect what you are trying to convey. For example, a student wrote:

The authors made no predictions regarding relationships in this exploratory study. What they did predict was the existence of a relationship between the independent and dependent variables (nondirectional hypotheses).

Well, which is it? Did the authors make predictions or did they not make predictions?

Another student wrote:

> The age in which women are becoming pregnant has both decreased and increased over the years in that we find more teenagers becoming pregnant as well as older couples attempting to start or continue a family.

After reading the sentence twice I understood the idea that the student was trying to convey; however, your goal is to write clearly so the reader does not have to make an effort to understand what you are trying to say. For example, the sentence above could have been written:

The pregnancy rate of adolescent and older women has increased over the past decade.

Show the Reader What You Mean

One of your primary goals in writing is to convey your thoughts and ideas to others. One giant obstacle to achieving this goal is that often the words that you use to convey your thoughts and ideas do not mean the same things to others. Consequently, it is usually a good idea to use examples to illustrate your points and show the reader what you are trying to convey. For example, in one paper a student wrote, "Clearly, the major features of the theory are described to the reader." I would have learned the major features of the theory and gotten the sense that the student knew the major features of the theory if she had followed the sentence above with an example of one of the major features that she said were described. For example, she might have written the sentence like this:

> The author does a good job of describing the major features of the theory. These features are symptom experience, symptom management, and symptom outcome.

Connect the Dots

While I have suggested that you use headings to structure your papers in nursing school, this does not mean that you will not have to pay attention to the continuity of your ideas. What I mean by continuity of ideas is that each sentence has to connect to the preceding sentence and each paragraph to the preceding paragraph so that you do not lose the reader. One way to avoid losing the reader is to include something from the previous sentence in the sentence that follows. For example, look at the italicized text in the sentences below:

> What I mean by continuity of ideas is that each sentence has to connect to the preceding sentence and each paragraph to the preceding paragraph so that you do not *lose the reader*. One way to avoid *losing the reader* is to include something from the previous sentence in the sentence that follows.

One of the difficulties in achieving an orderly presentation of ideas stems from the fact that you as the writer have a good idea of what you are trying to say. Consequently, in your proofreading it is very difficult to detect areas where your ideas do not flow in an orderly manner.

How do you improve the continuity of your ideas in your writing? Having others proofread your papers or, at the very least, having the paper read to you will help you become more alert to places where you may have lost the reader. In these areas you should expand your use of punctuation to change the pace of your writing. You also want to expand your use of transitional words such as: *consequently, in addition,* and *however* to make it easier for the reader to follow you.

Proofreading

The importance of proofreading your paper before submitting it cannot be overemphasized. This is especially true if you are submitting your paper electronically; most word-processing programs will identify such errors as double punctuation marks, misspelled words, and obvious grammatical errors. The errors that you did not bother to address before submitting your paper electronically will appear

Sidebar 10-1

Students for Whom English Is a Second Language

I have read many papers from students for whom English is a second language, and sometimes the grammar is so bad that I cannot even evaluate the paper. Most colleges and universities have resources such as writing labs for students who have difficulty with English or difficulty with written expression. Students should take advantage of these resources. Students who do not have access to writing labs need to find a classmate, peer, or tutor who can provide help with writing papers. While some nurses will spend little time with written expression, all nurses have to communicate ideas or information in writing at some time during their career; consequently, it is important that students be able to use proper grammar and sentence structure.

Cynthia Ayres, PhD, RN
Assistant Professor, College of Nursing
Rutgers, The State University of New Jersey

on your professor's screen when he or she opens up your paper on a computer. For example, a sentence like this one makes it clear that you performed no proofreading of your paper: "This research project was ethically stable but lacked a random opoulation sample." A paper that has obvious errors in spelling and formatting signals to the reader that there will probably be more significant problems in other areas of the paper as well. Moreover, I mentioned above that your professor would rather be doing something other than reading your paper, and the fact that you turned in a paper with little or no proofreading only generates more negative emotion in your professor.

In addition to using the grammar checking and spell checking features on the word-processing program that you use, print out your paper (or use print preview to conserve paper) to inspect your paper for glaring issues in formatting, such as errors in indentation or too much space between paragraphs. Most importantly, you need your paper read. If you have a friend or relative that you trust to proofread your paper, ask that person to proofread it. There is also a Speech option in Microsoft Word under "Tools" in which a computer voice reads your text aloud. You will be astounded at the number of errors you will pick up by simply taking the time to listen to what you wrote.

Sidebar 10-2

Get Feedback from Someone Outside of Nursing

One piece of advice that I have given nursing students about writing papers is to have a nonnursing peer read the paper before submitting it. Good writing is good writing, and if your prose is not clear to your nonnurse reader, it is probably not going to be clear to the faculty member who reads the paper and assigns your grade.

Jane Kurz, PhD, RN
Associate Professor,
Department of Nursing
Temple University

What Not to Do

In addition to putting time and energy into proofreading your papers before submitting them, you want to avoid several other steps that many students make.

Cutting and Pasting

One mistake many students make in writing papers involves taking excerpts from an article that they read and placing it into their paper. I have read papers that amount to nothing more than a few sentences by the student and excerpted texts from articles that the student references. Most of your professors will not be impressed with this technique of padding your paper. You would be better off in summarizing the main points of the author and trying to say something thoughtful regarding those points.

Listing

Another sure method to lower your grade on a paper is to include bulleted lists in your text. This commonly used technique looks like this (I have not corrected the spelling errors and formatting errors):

> Furtehrmore, this site also gave me both inborn and acuired causes of thrmobocyopenia.
>
> - Inborn causes
>   - Pancytopenias and thrombocytopenias
>   - Bone marrow infiltrates
>   - Rubella
>   - Maternal use of thiazide diuretics during pregnancy

This particular list ran on for three quarters of a page. The student could have easily rewritten the sentence to read, "Inborn causes of thrombocytopenia include pancytopenias and thrombocytopenias, bone marrow infiltrates, and rubella." This kind of ploy may fill up space in your paper, but it does not contribute to what you are getting out of nursing school or your grade.

Formatting Your Paper

The final section of this chapter covers formatting your paper. In high school and maybe in other college majors, your teachers probably did not focus too much on the size of your margins, how you cited references, or the font size you used. These formatting issues are of greater importance in nursing school and other academic settings. In most nursing schools the formatting system that is employed comes from the *Publication Manual of the American Psychological Association*, or APA. When I was in nursing school most of the faculty said that they enforced the APA format so that when students write for publication they will know how to format their papers. This rationale sounds good, but most students never write for publication. Emphasizing APA format in nursing school is akin to teaching students living in Florida how to drive in snowy conditions. It is not a bad thing for the students to know how to do, but it is unlikely that many of them will be driving in snowy conditions, and those who do can learn those skills when they need them.

It is not uncommon for APA format to count for 10% of your grade, and I have seen paper guidelines where it has accounted for 20%. You do not have to be a mathematician to know that simply formatting your paper appropriately can be the difference between an *A* and a *B*.

The complete guidelines for formatting manuscripts according to the APA are provided in the *Publication Manual of the American Psychological Association*, 5th edition, (2001). Appendix 10-A is a sample paper that has been formatted using APA. The next section reviews the basics of APA that you need to know and use in formatting your papers.

Title Page

The format of the title page varies by educational institution, but according to the APA manual your title page should include a running head for publication, title, and your name. If you are using Microsoft Word, here is how to create your title page:

- Aligned left at the top of your paper type: Running Head: Soybean Protein (all capital letters, no more than 50 characters).
- Use the Enter key to space down to about 4″ (stay in the upper half of the page). In uppercase and lowercase letters, type your title. If you are using Microsoft Word, go under Format→Paragraph→Alignment→Center to center your title.
- The Running Head is an abbreviated title that appears at the top of all the pages of your paper. To create the running head using Microsoft Word go under View→Header and Footer. A header box will appear. Use the ruler or Format→Paragraph→Alignment→Right to right justify your header. Type your running head into the header box: Common Cold. Use the space bar to create 10 spaces, and then use the Header and Footer ruler box and type #. You now have a running head.

Spacing, Fonts, and Margins

Use double line spacing. If you are using Microsoft Word, go under Format →Paragraph→Line spacing→Double.

Do not get fancy with the font. Use 12-pt Times Roman or 12-pt Courier. If you are using Microsoft Word, go under Format→Font→Font = Times Roman or Courier Size = 12.

Make the margins a uniform 1 inch (2.54 cm) at the top, bottom, left, and right of every page. If you are using Microsoft Word, go under File→Page Setup→Margins.

Paraphrasing and Summarizing

Authors have two options when citing borrowed material that has been summarized or paraphrased. A signal statement containing the author's last name followed by the publication date in parentheses can precede the borrowed material:

> Atkins and Hart (2003) found that youth in urban neighborhoods with high levels of poverty were less likely than their counterparts in less impoverished and suburban neighborhoods to perform community service.

The same borrowed material can be acknowledged with the author and date in parentheses following the borrowed material:

> Youth in urban neighborhoods with high levels of poverty were less likely than their counterparts in less impoverished and suburban neighborhoods to perform community service (Atkins & Hart, 2003).

In both cases the past tense with signal verbs is used: *found, reported, showed*. Notice when citing two authors following the borrowed material, an ampersand (&) is used to join the two authors' names in the parentheses.

A Source by Three to Five Authors

When borrowed material comes from a source with more than two authors (but fewer than six authors), cite each of the authors the first time that source is cited. However, in subsequent citations, include only the last name of the first author followed by *et al.* (not in italic font) and the year of the publication:

> Resilient children were more likely to engage in prosocial behaviors like sharing than over-controlled and under-controlled children (Atkins, Hart, & Donnelly, 2005).

In subsequent citations it would be: Atkins et al. (2005).

A Source by Six or More Authors

If the source of the borrowed material has six or more authors, only the last name of the first author is cited followed by *et al.* (not in italic font) and the year of the publication.

In the reference list the first six authors are cited by last name and initials (e.g., Robert L. Atkins = Atkins, R. L.). When a source is cited that has more than six authors the remaining authors are identified as *et al.*

Groups as Authors

When borrowing material from groups of authors where corporate, government, or association names serve as the author names, the group name should be spelled out the first time that it is cited in the text:

> National estimates based on Emergency Department records from 2003 indicate that there were 339,697 assault-related nonfatal injuries for youth between the ages of 12 and 17 years of age (Centers for Disease Control, 2005).

Subsequent citations of this source may refer to the Centers for Disease Control (CDC, 2005).

Direct Quotation

In some cases authors choose to borrow material that they have quoted verbatim. As with paraphrased or summarized material, the author must include the author's last name, date of publication, and, in addition, the page number at the end of the quotation:

> Reflection is a component of virtually all service-learning programs. Writing about reflection, Eyler and Giles (1999) referred to it as the "link that ties student experiences in the community to academic learning" (p. 171).

The author's last name, date of publication, and page number can also follow the quotation:

> Reflection is a component of virtually all service-learning programs and has been referred to it as the "link that ties student experiences in the community to academic learning" (Eyler & Giles, 1999, p. 171).

Reference List

The author-date format of sources in the APA guidelines makes it easy for readers to locate the complete entry in the reference list. The reference list contains complete publication information for each of the sources cited in a paper. The references are listed on a separate page at the end of your paper. If you have figures or tables as part of your paper, the references precede these pages.

Title, Spacing, and Order of References

At the top of the page that contains the references, the word *References* should be centered.

The line spacing of the reference section is double-space as with the main body of the paper.

Alphabetize your references by the last name of the first author or the group name. If you use more than one work by the same author the earliest reference is listed first.

Hanging Indentation

The first line of each reference is flush with the left margin, and the subsequent lines are indented about one half inch. (If you are using Microsoft Word: Format →Special→Hanging). A reference to a journal article would look like this:

Mainous, A. G., Hueston, W. J., & Clark, J. R. (1996). Antibiotics and upper respiratory infection: Do some folks think there is a cure for the common cold? *Journal of Family Practice, 42,* 357–361.

Format of Entries in Reference List

Names of Authors

As reflected in the citation above, authors are listed in the reference section by their last name and first two initials. When there is more than one author an ampersand (&) is used.

Publication Date

The date of the publication follows the author(s) names and is placed in parentheses followed by a period.

Title of Work

The title of the article (in journals, magazines, scholarly newsletters, online periodicals), title of work (book, online document), or title of chapter (book chapter) follows the publication date. When formatting citations of articles, chapters, and online periodicals, the title of the work is followed by the title of the periodical, book in which the chapter appeared, or the title of the online periodical.

Publication Information

When citing a journal article, the title of the journal, the volume number, and the inclusive page numbers of the journal article are included in the citation. For a book citation the publisher location and publisher name follows the title of the book. For a book chapter the names of the book editors (initials of editors' first names and then last name), the title of the book, the inclusive page numbers, the location, and the publisher are included.

Specific Formats of Citations

The general formats for specific types of citations are listed here:

Journal Article

Smith, J., Jones, D., & Doe, J. (publication year). Title of article. *Title of Journal, volume number,* page numbers.

Book

Smith, J., Jones, D., & Doe, J. (publication year). *Title of work.* Location: Publisher.

Chapter in Edited Book

Smith, J., Jones, D., & Doe, J. (publication year). Title of chapter. In J. Smith, D. Jones, & J. Doe (Eds.), *Title of book* (pp. xx–xx). Location: Publisher.

Internet Periodical

Smith, J., Jones, D., & Doe, J. (publication year). Title of article. *Title of Internet Periodical, volume number,* page numbers. Retrieved August 1, 2007, from source.

Internet Document

Smith, J. (publication year). *Title of work.* Retrieved August 1, 2007, from source (e.g., http://www.internet.org)

No problem right? A little attention to formatting the references correctly improves the look of your paper and earns you some points that might otherwise be deducted.

If you are having trouble figuring out how to properly format your references and citations in your text, there are some great resources on the Internet. One resource, Landmarks Son of Citation Machine (http://citationmachine.net/index.php), will format your references in APA for you. All you have to do is enter the information (e.g., author's last name, page numbers) and paste the reference generated on the site into your document.

Conclusion

I do not offer myself as an expert on writing, and the recommendations offered in this book on improving one's writing in nursing school are only a place to begin. I chose to focus on these areas for improvement based on what has stood out from my experiences of reading papers in nursing school. It would be easy to devote an entire book to improving one's writing and, in fact, there are some excellent books on writing that will help you improve your writing (for example, Michael Harvey's *The Nuts and Bolts of College Writing* and the companion Web site: http://nutsandbolts. washcoll.edu/nb-home.html). There are also Internet resources such as the University of Toronto's Advice on Academic Writing: http://www.utoronto.ca/writing/advise. html and the OWL at Purdue University: http://owl.english.purdue.edu/owl/

In the appendix I have provided a sample paper submitted by Lynne Verderese, an exemplary nursing student from a class I taught. Mrs. Verderese was kind enough to permit me to critique her paper. Overall, the paper exemplifies a well-written student paper in terms of formatting, organization, and coherence; however, as I have learned, there is almost always room for improvement in writing. For the purposes of this book, I have looked at the paper very critically and commented on areas in the student's paper which are done well (+ +) and areas that need improvement (PROBLEMS). Use the strengths and weaknesses identified in this paper to think about how you can improve the papers you submit.

References

Publication manual of the American Psychological Association (5th ed.). (2001). Washington, DC: American Psychological Association.

Melnyk, B. M., & Fineholt-Overholt, E. (2005). *Evidence-based practice in nursing and healthcare: A guide to best practice.* Philadelphia: Lippincott.

APPENDIX 10-A

Sample Paper with Critique

Running Head: Soybean Protein

> **COMMENT:**
> See instructions on formatting Running head, headers, and title page in Chapter 10.

Research Critique:
Effect of Soybean Protein
on Blood Pressure

> **COMMENT:**
> APA: Because this paper is not being submitted for review in a journal, this title page is acceptable.

Lynne S. Verderese

Rutgers, The State University
of New Jersey

Effect of Soybean Protein
on Blood Pressure

> **COMMENT:**
> APA: Title of paper typed in first line.

Blood pressure refers to the force of blood as it pushes against the arteries. When this force of blood is greater than normal, referred to as hypertension, there are a number of complications that may occur such as heart disease, heart attack, congestive heart failure, stroke, kidney failure, peripheral artery disease, and aortic aneurysms. A range of interventions to reduce blood pressure have been tested in clinical trials (e.g., weight loss, exercise, alcohol restriction, sodium reduction, and potassium supplementation). The effect of nutritional intervention, specifically dietary macronutrients on blood pressure, has not been well studied. Epidemiological studies observed an inverse relationship between dietary protein and blood pressure.

> **COMMENT:**
> ++ While the paper is not about the complications of hypertension, the student provided some background and significance to establish why this topic is important.

In this paper I will provide a critique of a study in which investigators examined the relationship between dietary protein and blood pressure. This study, entitled: *Effect of Soybean Protein on Blood Pressure,* was published in a 2005 issue of the Annals of Internal Medicine.

> **COMMENT:**
> ++. This is a good transition. Note that the first sentence of this paragraphs relates to the last sentence of the preceding paragraph.

> **COMMENT:**
> The author does a good job of orienting the reader as to what is to come.

Research Problem

The focus of this research study was to measure the effect of soybean protein supplementation on blood pressure in patients with pre-hypertension or stage 1 hypertension. A specific hypothesis was not articulated in the introduction, method, or discussion sections of this research study and the value of reduction in blood pressure required for a level of significance was not enumerated until the statistical analysis section. The more general problem statement was presented as previous observational studies suggest that higher intake of vegetable protein is associated with lower blood pressures.

> **COMMENT:**
> ++. The author makes good use of headings throughout the paper to orient the reader. These headings are taken directly from the guidelines that the student received.

Literature Review

The list of references for this research study was extensive; however, the initial discussion of the referred clinical trials was too terse to provide adequate understanding of the previous research in this area. This study states, "the few clinical trials that examined the effect of an increased intake of dietary protein on blood pressure produced conflicting results" (He et al., 2005, p. 5). The previous trials that were studied had either small sample sizes or only single blood pressure measurements. A study by Stamler (1996) was referenced in this study. Stamler (1996) observed an inverse relationship of dietary protein consumption with blood pressure. While there were 10,020 subjects enrolled in the study authored by Stamler, this study was not a randomized, controlled clinical trial.

Later in the discussion of the statistical analysis section of the study, a more thorough presentation of previous research in this area was compared to this study. One previous study by Washburn, Burke, Morgan and Anthony (1999) compared the effect of consumption of 20g of soybean protein with that of 20g of carbohydrates on cardiovascular risks on 51 perimenopausal women. The sample size in this previous study was very small but did demonstrate a statistically significant effect on blood pressure. The researchers wanted to extend this previous research using a larger, more diverse sample and a randomized, controlled trial.

Research Design

The research study was a randomized, double-blind, controlled trial designed to test the efficacy of 40g of isolated soybean protein supplementation per day in lowering blood pressure in patients with prehypertension or stage 1 hypertension. The control group received 40g of complex carbohydrate per day. Both groups consumed these

---

COMMENT:

PROBLEM. Anthropomorphism or attributing human characteristics to animals or inanimate sources is a common error in writing: "The study states". . .a study does not have a voice so it cannot state. It would be better to rephrase this sentence to read something like: He and colleagues wrote,. . .

COMMENT:

APA formatting. Quotation of fewer than 40 words. Author, year, specific page.

COMMENT:

APA formatting. Within the same paragraph you need to include the year only in the first reference to the study.

COMMENT:

PROBLEM. As a reader it is not clear what *this* refers to. Is the author referring to the Stamler article or the He article?

COMMENT:

PROBLEM. Again, it is not clear who the researchers are. It would be better to write He et al. (2005).

supplement cookies for 12 weeks. Blood pressure measurements were taken at baseline, at six weeks, and at 12 weeks, using random-zero sphygmomanometers.

A study dietitian counseled the participants on reduction of food intake to compensate for the additional 40g of nutrients. The participants were also instructed to maintain their usual level of activity, alcohol intake, and dietary sodium. The counseling attempted to mitigate any mediating or confounding factors that might affect the dependent variable, blood pressure.

Sample

Three clinical centers in the People's Republic of China participated in the trial. The participants were men and women 35 to 65 years of age with an average systolic blood pressure of 130 to 150 mmHg, a diastolic blood pressure of 80 to 99 mmHg, or both over an average of 9 readings (He et al., 2005). Excluded patients included those that had used anti-hypertensive medication in the previous two months or those that had other co-existing life-threatening illnesses or psychiatric disease. A sample of 302 patients met the eligibility requirements and was randomly assigned to the treatment or control group.

Data Collection

The researchers collected information on medical history, medication use, alcohol consumption, and physical activity at baseline. Trained study staff members measured blood pressure from the right arm after the patient was seated quietly for 5 minutes. Three blood pressure measurements were obtained at each of 3 screening visits: before intervention, at 6 weeks, and at 12 weeks after randomization. Weight, height, and waist circumference were measured and body mass index (BMI) was calculated based on a standard formula. A 24-hour dietary recall was conducted at the three screening visits.

Data Analysis

This trial was designed to provide a β value of 0.2 (power of 80%) in detecting a 3.0mm Hg reduction in systolic pressure and a 2.0mm Hg reduction in diastolic pressure at a significance level of 0.05. All statistical tests were two-tailed. The attrition rate in this study was low, providing a large sample that completed the study. A total of 92.7% of participants in the soybean supplementation group and 90.1 of the control group completed the study.

At the 6-week visit, the average change in systolic blood pressure was –8.6 mm Hg (SD 9.4) in the soybean protein group and –5.9 mm Hg (SD 11.2) in the control group. The net difference in systolic blood pressure was –2.66 mm Hg for the soybean group compared with the control group. At the 12-week visit, the average change in systolic blood pressure was –13.0 mm Hg (SD 9.7) in the soybean group and –8.7 mm Hg (SD 9.0) in the control group. The net difference in systolic blood pressure was –4.31 mm Hg for the soybean group compared with the control group. The net difference in diastolic blood pressure for the soybean protein group compared with the control group at 6 weeks and 12 weeks was –1.17 mm Hg and –2.76 mm Hg respectively (He et al., 2005).

The effects of the soybean intervention were less pronounced in the prehypertensive group than in those with hypertension. Only the results

COMMENT:

PROBLEM. These sentences could be written over to read: "The attrition rate in this study was low. A total of 92.7% of participants in the soybean supplementation group and 90.1 of the control group completed the study."

for the hypertensive group were significant for both systolic and diastolic blood pressure. No adverse side effects were experienced as a result of the soybean supplementation.

The effect data was further categorized by subgroups. For the subgroups by gender or age, no statistical difference in effect based on the subgroup was documented. For the subgroups of overweight (BMI > 25 kg/m^2) vs. non-overweight a reduction in systolic blood pressure of -3.59 mm Hg vs. -6.49 mm Hg was reported. Therefore, the intervention was 1.8 times more effective on non-overweight people as overweight people.

Conclusions

This study, compared with previous studies on soybean protein effects on blood pressure, had the largest sample size and several measurements of blood pressure. The results indicated that soybean supplementation reduced both systolic and diastolic blood pressure. The blood pressure reduction was documented for men and women, young and old, normal weight and overweight participants allowing for applicability across the population. To date, soybean protein supplementation has presented greater reduction in blood pressure than other currently recommended lifestyle modifications, except for the DASH diet (Appel et al., 1997). Therefore, soy protein may be recommended as one effective approach in reducing blood pressure in patients with stage 1 hypertension.

Limitations and Application

One of the limitations defined in the study was the inability to control the patient's daily food intake. The consumption of the protein or complex carbohydrate cookies in lieu of saturated fats in the

COMMENT:
++ The use of *Therefore* is a good transition device.

COMMENT:
++ The author did not neglect to write a conclusion.

COMMENT:
PROBLEM. This sentence is a little clunky. I think it would read better if the author had written: "The critiqued study by He and colleagues was the largest and best controlled study of the effects of soybean protein on blood pressure."

COMMENT:
PROBLEM. Poor word choice. I think the author meant *generalizability* rather than *applicability*.

COMMENT:
PROBLEM. Poor word choice. I think the author meant to write "has resulted in a greater reduction in blood pressure."

COMMENT:
PROBLEM. I think the author could have used a transitional sentence to ease the reader into this section of the paper. A sentence such as:
"There were several limitations to the study that I critiqued."

COMMENT:
PROBLEM. The presentation of ideas in this paragraph is not orderly. The author brings up a limitation and then returns to a discussion of soybean protein supplementation.

diet produced a greater reduction in blood pressure than the difference between the intervention and control group. Therefore, a patient would benefit from both the reduction in saturated fat and the soybean protein supplementation.

Another limitation to the study was the regional sample. The Chinese diet consists largely of vegetable protein sources while the American diet is mostly meat protein. The applicability of the blood pressure reduction using vegetable protein supplementation in the United States is not clear. The genetic and dietary differences in the two populations may not yield the same results.

A variable that was not controlled in this study was smoking vs. non-smoking participants. About 21% of the soybean group and 16% of the control group were smokers. A completely non-smoking sample should have been selected to remove the moderating effect on the outcome. Since individual results for smokers and non-smokers were not provided, the effect of this additional variable was unknown.

This quantitative study provided a randomized, double-blind controlled trial that produced findings suggesting that the increased intake of soybean protein may play a role in treating stage 1 hypertension. Further studies in U.S. populations and studies that help determine whether isoflavones in soy or the protein are the source of the blood pressure reduction should be conducted.

> **COMMENT:**
>
> PROBLEM. The author probably needs to cue the reader that she is still discussing limitations by writing the sentence like this: "A third limitation to the study was that the researchers did not control for cigarette smoking in the study design."

> **COMMENT:**
>
> PROBLEM. This sentence does not make sense. I think the author meant to write: "A variable that was not adequately controlled in this study was smoking." In addition, random assignment makes it unnecessary to control for smoking.

> **COMMENT:**
>
> PROBLEM. This sentence could be written simpler:
> "The findings from this well-designed randomized controlled study suggest that the increased intake of soybean protein may play a role in decreasing stage 1 hypertension."

References

Appel, L. J., Moore, T. J., Obarzanek, E., Vollmer, W. M., Svetsky, L. P., Sacks, F. M., et al. (1997). A clinical trial of the effects of dietary patterns on blood pressure. DASH Collaborative Research Group. *New England Journal of Medicine, 336,* 1117–1124.

He, J., Gu, D., Wu, X., Chen, J., Duan, X., Chen, J., & Whelton, P. K. (2005). Effect of soybean protein on blood pressure. *Annals of Internal Medicine, 143,* 1–10.

Stamler, J., Elliott, P., Kesteloot, H., Nichols, R., Claeys, G., Dyer, A. R., et al. (1996). Inverse relation of dietary protein markers with blood pressure. Findings for 10,020 men and women in the INTERSALT study. *Circulation, 94,* 1629–1634.

Washburn, S., Burke, G. I., Morgan, T., & Anthony, M., (1999). Effect of soy protein supplementation on serum lipoproteins, blood pressure, and menopausal symptoms in perimenopausal women. *Menopause, 6,* 7–13.

COMMENT:

APA: See Chapter 10 for instructions on how to format Reference section.

ELEVEN

A Short Chapter on Academic Dishonesty

A short chapter on academic dishonesty has been included in this book because few things runs more counter to the goals of this book than cheating. As emphasized throughout this book, your goal as a student in nursing school is to get the most out of your nursing school education so that you can be the best possible nurse for the patients and families who will rely on your knowledge and skills. Every act of academic dishonesty is a shortcut that diminishes what one gets out of nursing school and limits your ability to be the best possible healthcare provider. Surprisingly, there is some evidence to suggest that forms of academic dishonesty, like cheating on an exam, result in lower (not higher) grades (Whitley & Keith-Spiegel, 2001). Thus, cheaters pay at least two costs: they have failed to master the material, and their academic dishonesty has resulted in lower grades.

Unfortunately, these costs are not enough to dissuade many students from cheating. Indeed there is some anecdotal and empirical evidence to suggest that a growing number of high school and college students are engaging in academic dishonesty. Consonant with these findings are surveys that suggest academic dishonesty has become more socially acceptable (Harris, 2001). In fact, a recent study of more than 5,000 graduate school students in the United

States and Canada found that about half of the students (56% of graduate students in business school) admitted to engaging in some form of academically dishonest behavior such as plagiarizing (McCabe, Trevino, & Butterfield, 2001).

There are many forms of academic dishonesty, and most students probably know that flagrantly dishonest acts such as buying a paper off of the Internet and submitting it as one's own work goes against the academic code. However, there are more subtle forms of academic dishonesty (e.g., recycling a paper that you received credit for in a prior class) that some students may not be entirely sure constitute academic dishonesty. Of course, a good rule of thumb to go by is that: if you are doing something you think may be unethical or academically dishonest or something that might be giving you an unfair advantage over your classmates, then it probably is a violation of the academic code. The discussion in this chapter will cover the categories of academic dishonesty and hopefully clear up any confusion on what constitutes academic dishonesty.

Cheating

Although all forms of academic dishonesty can be considered cheating, in most academic settings cheating refers to the covert or unauthorized use of materials, information, or study aids in an academic assignment such as an exam or homework assignment. These forms of cheating include the purchase of papers on the Internet, stealing exams, and recording answers or information to be used during the exam on crib sheets, cell phones, or parts of the body. Cheating also includes assistance from others that is voluntary (e.g., Student A whispering the answer for question #35 to Student B) or involuntary (e.g., Student A looking over Student B's shoulder to determine what Student B chose for question #35).

Fabrication

Another form of academic dishonesty involves the falsification or invention of information in an academic assignment. Instances of fabrication that occur in the academic (and real-world) settings include the generation of bogus data in order to get the desired results and the generation of false sources of information for research papers or other assignments. Acts of fabrication also include signing an attendance sheet for another student. An especially unethical and dangerous form of fabrication, unique to the clinical setting, involves the documentation of invented data (e.g., blood pressure, urine output, etc.) in a patient's record. Although it may seem minor to document that a patient's vital signs were stable when, in fact, the vital signs were not assessed, this is a slippery slope, and most clinical instructors are especially vigilant in identifying and punishing students who would engage in this type of dishonest behavior. A student who fabricates vital signs may become a nurse who documents that a medication was given when it was not, which endangers the patient and discredits the nursing profession.

Facilitating Academic Dishonesty

Even when students themselves do not benefit from academic dishonesty, facilitating or assisting others to engage in academic dishonesty is a violation of the academic code. For example, when Student A whispers the answer for question #35 to Student B or when Student A helps Student B to break into the school and steal an exam, Student A is as guilty of academic dishonesty as Student B.

Plagiarism

Plagiarism is the use of another's words or ideas without properly crediting that source. While the Internet has made it much easier to plagiarize the work of others, it has also made it easier for faculty to identify plagiarism from Internet sources. For example, faculty who suspect plagiarism can use the Google search engine to search a few words from a student's paper enclosed by quotation marks or they can use Internet services such as www.turnitin.com to have an entire paper scanned for plagiarized passages. Most institutions have clearly defined consequences for plagiarism and other forms of cheating ranging from a failing grade on an assignment to dismissal from the nursing program. Obviously, getting the most out of nursing school is predicated on the assumption that you remain a student in good standing. Consequently, it is in your best interest to avoid intentionally or unintentionally using the work of another without properly crediting that source. Discussed in the section below are some of the most common forms of plagiarism and how to avoid them.

Cutting and Pasting

While cutting and pasting has been discussed above as a bad form of writing, it is also a form of plagiarism when it involves cutting words from one source (e.g., a document found on the Internet) and pasting those words into your paper. Consider the sentence below taken from Von Ah, Kang, and Carpenter (2007):

> Understanding how optimism and satisfaction with social support relate to the psychological stress of breast cancer diagnosis and surgical treatment will greatly improve our ability to design tailored interventions to address the demands these women face.

Even if this sentence expresses your thoughts precisely, you commit plagiarism if you insert it into your paper and do not place quotations around it and properly cite Von Ah and colleagues. Of course, writing assignments are given to evaluate critical thinking skills and the ability to express oneself, not to assess your ability to string together quotations from different sources; consequently, you run the risk of receiving a failing grade for your paper if it amounts to nothing more than a series of quotations from different sources. Moreover, you could be plagiarizing, and you are probably violating a variety of intellectual property and copyright laws by submitting a paper with a series of quotations without citations.

Inappropriate Paraphrasing

While most students know that it is plagiarism to place a sentence directly from another source into their paper without citing the source, it is also unacceptable to shuffle the words around and not cite the source. Let's look at the passage from Von Ah et al. (2007) again:

> Our ability to design interventions tailored to the needs of women will be enhanced as we understand how optimism and satisfaction with social support connect to the psychological stress of breast cancer diagnosis and surgical treatment.

As you can see, the words have been moved around but the idea is the same and Von Ah et al. have not been cited.

One way to avoid plagiarism would be to include something like this: The effectiveness of interventions for women dealing with breast cancer diagnosis and surgical treatment will be improved as researchers and clinicians better understand the extent to which optimism and satisfaction with social support mediate the association between stress and immune response (Von Ah, Kang, & Carpenter, 2007).

The idea of Von et al. has been cited and you have paraphrased what the authors said.

Multiple Submissions

Most students understand that if they obtain a paper written by another (e.g., sibling, friend, or some anonymous source on the Internet) and submit it for credit in a class as their own, they have committed plagiarism. However, another form of plagiarism is to recycle, or resubmit, a paper that you had used for credit in a previous course. While you may really like the paper that you wrote for a previous course and you may feel that it meets the requirements for another course, you are committing plagiarism if you resubmit a paper. Not only is this behavior academically dishonest, but the probability that you will get away with this tactic is low. Believe it or not, faculty in most nursing programs do know what assignments are given in other courses, and your professor will have little difficulty in determining if you are attempting to re-cycle a paper and, while the educator may not formally report this as an academic offense, you can be sure that this maneuver will lower your grade. While most edu-cators do not want to read your papers, they do expect that you will write a "fresh" one for their class. The number of students who have told me that "a professor in an-other class gave me a better grade for this paper" suggests to me that many students are unaware that this type of recycling is unethical and dishonest.

How to Avoid Plagiarism

Besides being knowledgeable of the proper scholarly conventions involved in writ-ing papers (information can be found in the Web sites listed at the end of this chap-ter), one of the most effective steps students can take to avoid plagiarism is to start the writing process well in advance of the deadline. While I have only anecdotal ev-idence to support this recommendation, I have found that students seem to get "caught up" in plagiarism—rather than making a conscious decision at the beginning of their academic careers to act unethically—as they try to overcome the challenge of pro-ducing a good academic product when they have not budgeted enough time. As dis-cussed in Chapter 13, time management is crucial in nursing school and the profession of nursing.

Interfering with the Access of Others to Information or Material

The final category of academic dishonesty is actions taken by students aimed at blocking or denying the academic or scholarly pursuits of others. In contrast to the other forms of academic dishonesty that have been discussed in which students focus on improving their grades by taking actions that put them at an advantage, students who engage in forms of academic dishonesty that involve interfering seek to improve their grade by "sticking it to the other guy." These kinds of acts include concealing, destroying, or damaging laboratory or library materials to deprive others of the use of these materials.

Conclusion

The institutional consequences for individuals who engage in academic dishonesty depend on a number of factors such as the nature of the offense and whether the individual has a history of academic dishonesty. In most cases, penalties for infractions of the academic code range from a zero on the academic exercise to expulsion from the educational institution. Of course, these consequences will only be exacted if one is caught engaging in academic dishonesty. There are at least three other hidden consequences—perhaps more serious consequences—that can occur regardless of whether the individual is caught.

Consequences to the Individual

The first consequence is that there is some evidence that students who cheat damage their moral compass and begin down a path that extends beyond their educational setting. This may be why students who do not abide by an honor code in school are more likely than their counterparts who did follow an honor code in school to engage in dishonest behavior in the workplace (McCabe et al., 2001). This finding is especially troubling in nursing because moral integrity and ethical behavior are the foundation upon which the profession is built, and the public trusts nurses more than any other profession to be honest and ethical (Artz, 2006).

Consequences for Other Students

The other consequence of academic dishonesty has to do with how each act of academic dishonesty degrades the learning environment. This degradation of the learning environment begins with a loss of trust among students and faculty, and every member of the learning community, honest and dishonest, suffers as trust is replaced by suspicion and cynicism. Students and faculty wonder whether the accomplishments of other students are due to hard work or academic dishonesty. As the learning environment creeps downward, students who might not otherwise engage in academic dishonest behavior become cynical and may rationalize that cheating is normal and acceptable behavior (McCabe et al., 2001).

Consequences for the Faculty

It is pretty safe to assert that most educators have a deep dislike of dishonest behavior in their students and are vigilant in their efforts to identify cheating by their students. As noted, faculty in nursing school are probably even more vigilant in identifying cheaters because graduates of our programs will go directly into jobs where their character and honesty influence the health and well-being of others (Bellack, 2004). For example, when a nurse falsely reports that a treatment or medication was given, the health of the patient is jeopardized. Consequently, when academic dishonesty is encountered in nursing programs, faculty have to allocate resources that would otherwise go to advising students or improving the curriculum to safeguarding against academic dishonesty by writing multiple versions of exams and proctoring exams to prevent students from cheating. This redirection of faculty resources further degrades the learning environment.

Consequences for the Institution

If enough students begin to engage in academic dishonesty, the learning community may degrade to a point where others outside of the learning community (e.g., employers, accrediting agencies potential students, and potential faculty) become aware of what is happening within the learning institution. At the very least this awareness diminishes the value of the degree earned at that institution and the institution develops a reputation for lacking integrity. This type of reputation persists at the Air Force Academy, which has endured five cheating scandals over the past 40 years. In the latest cheating scandal, which happened in February 2007, the Air Force Academy investigated allegations of cheating by 28 freshmen. According to the academy's spokesperson, Johnny Whitaker, the academy's superintendent asked the cadets in a speech "Is this the kind of institution that we want to be? Honor is the heart of what we do" (Cooperman, 2007). Honor is also at the heart of nursing.

Web-Based Information on Plagiarism and Academic Dishonesty

Avoiding Plagiarism. Handout from Purdue University Online Writing Lab (OWL), West Lafayette. http://owl.english.purdue.edu/owl/resource/589/01/.

A Guide to Library Research: How to Write a Better Paper. Developed by Rutgers University Library, New Jersey. http://www.libraries.rutgers.edu/rul/libs/robeson_lib/libres.html

How Not to Plagiarize. Developed by the University of Toronto, Toronto, Canada. http://www.utoronto.ca/writing/plagsep.html.

References

Artz, M. (2006). Ask not what nursing can do for you: Nurses have a lot of power. *American Journal of Nursing, 106,* 91.

Bellack, J. P. (2004). Why plagiarism matters. *Journal of Nursing Education, 43,* 527–528.

Cooperman, A. (2007, February 10). Air Force Academy probes alleged cheating by cadets. *Washington Post,* A03.

Harris, R. A. (2001). *The plagiarism handbook.* Los Angeles: Pyrczak.

McCabe, D. L., Trevino, L. K., & Butterfield, K. D. (2001). Cheating in academic institutions: A decade of research. *Ethics & Behavior, 11,* 219–232.

Von Ah, D., Kang, D. H., & Carpenter, J. S. (2007). Stress, optimism, and social support: Impact on immune responses in breast cancer. *Research in Nursing & Health, 30,* 72–83.

Whitley, B. E., & Keith-Spiegel, P. (2001). *Academic dishonesty: An educator's guide.* Princeton: Lawrence Erlbaum Associates.

TWELVE

Getting the Most Out of Clinical Coursework

A substantial portion of learning in nursing school occurs in the clinical setting. The clinical practice component in most nursing school curriculums is designed to complement what is learned in the theory course and the nursing skills labs. While the clinical placement varies by institution, in general, students are placed in hospitals, clinics, public health offices, and community agencies. In this chapter, an overview of the clinical component of nursing school is provided and suggestions are given for making the most of the clinical experience in nursing school.

Brief History of Clinical Experience

Prior to the 1960s, most nurses received their professional education in nursing schools that were affiliated with hospitals. In these nursing schools nursing students were trained through a hospital-based apprenticeship. During this apprenticeship, young women (they were essentially all young, unmarried women) lived within the hospital for a period ranging from 6 months to 3 years and were trained to be nurses by practicing nursing skills on patients in the hospital (Leighow, 1996). While nursing and nursing education have changed a great deal over the past 40 years, the clinical nursing education component of most modern nursing programs retains some of the characteristics of the hospital-based apprenticeship system of nursing training. For example, similar to the hospital-based apprenticeship system, students are placed in acute clinical settings, usually hospitals, where they are supervised by clinical faculty in providing care to one to three patients (Tanner, 2006).

Sidebar 12-1

Anticipatory Guidance for Nursing School Students

There are a number of experiences that you are going to face as a nursing school student and as a new nurse that will be easier to handle if you are prepared for them to occur. Here are a few of them and suggestions on how to handle these experiences:

1. *Healthcare is always changing, and you are going to always be asked to make changes.* Often in nursing, especially in the hospital setting, it seems that as soon as you are used to one way of doing things (e.g., charting, doing a procedure, dividing patient assignments, and entering orders), you are asked to adopt a new way of doing the same thing. For a number of reasons, most of us (us being humans not just nurses) resist change. I also dislike change, but in my career as a nurse I have found that it is better in the long run when I take a step back, think about the big picture, and give the change a chance to work. I remember when I was a new nurse and the unit I was on decided to change from "district nursing" to "primary nursing." I, with many of my colleagues, resisted the change but the change to primary nursing was one of the best things to happen on that floor while I was there.

2. *Just because someone is a healthcare professional does not mean they always act professionally.* There are going to be times in your nursing school education or your nursing career that a faculty member, fellow nursing student, or healthcare professional colleague (e.g., nurse, physician) acts unprofessionally. It may be that someone in the educational or work setting blows up at you and says something inappropriate in anger. Perhaps they did not like something that you did or something that you did not do. In these situations it is important to take a step back and assess before taking action. Use what you learned in your nursing school education about working with patients. Remember that just because you are dealing with someone who is not in the "sick role" does not mean that the interpersonal skills that you employ in working with patients will be unproductive. You would not take it personally if a patient reacted unreasonably and, in the same way, you should not necessarily take it personally if a colleague has a bad-tempered response to you. As you will have learned by the end of your nursing education, many times an

individual who expresses anger may be reacting to a stressful situation by directing their anger at you. In deciding how to respond try to use your nursing skills to look past the anger, and remember, while your colleague's response may have been unprofessional, you want to remain professional.

3. *You may come to find that the position you have chosen and you believed was perfect for you is not perfect for you.* One of the best things about nursing is that, as a nurse, you have such a wide array of choices in terms of where you work (e.g., hospital, community), when you work (e.g., days, evenings, weekends), and the type of work you do as a nurse (e.g., medical-surgical, OR, pediatrics). Consequently, as I tell all of my students, if you don't like your job in nursing go find one that suits you better. Each job provides different opportunities and challenges and, especially with the nursing shortage, there is no reason to stay in a job that does not fit your needs.

4. *It will take at least 18 months and a day for you to feel like you are somewhat competent as a nurse.* In the first year and a half of your work as a registered nurse everything that you encounter is new. After about a year and a half you might finally come across some clinical problem that is familiar and you feel comfortable in handling because you dealt with it before. When that happens you may finally start to feel like you know what you are doing as a nurse.

Laurie Karmel, MSN, RN
Clinical Instructor, College of Nursing
Rutgers, The State University of New Jersey

What to Expect During Clinical Experience

Clinical Times

In most nursing schools, to complete the clinical component for each course students are required to participate in clinical 2 days a week (e.g., Tuesday and Thursday) for two 6-hour sessions. Depending on the program, the clinical times may be evenings or weekends. The clinical sessions for each course last 6–12 weeks.

Clinical Uniforms

Most schools of nursing have established dress codes. While many students bemoan the dress code, it benefits students in at least two ways. First, there is evidence to suggest that dressing in a professional manner improves one's rapport and working relationship with patients, families, and clinical staff (Mangum, Garrison, Lind, Thackeray, & Wyatt, 1991; Mangum, Garrison, Lind, & Hilton, 1997). Second, the nursing school uniform identifies you as a student to clinical staff, patients, and families. For example, if the clinical staff knows you are a student they may be more likely to share an interesting learning opportunity with you, and clinical staff may be less likely to ask you to do something that you are not qualified to do in an emergency situation (e.g., administer medications during a code). This dress code usually requires students to wear a uniform (e.g., white pants or knee-length white skirt, a uniform short-sleeved blouse, a long-sleeved short lab coat, white pantyhose or socks, and white shoes) during clinical with a patch on the jacket identifying the school of nursing the student is affiliated with. Most nursing school dress codes also include restrictions on sneakers and clogs, artificial nails (which have been shown to be contaminated with germs that cause infections in patients [Hedderwick, McNeil, Lyons, & Kauffman, 2000; McNeil, Foster, Hedderwick, & Kauffman, 2001; Moolenaar et al., 2000]), long fingernails, heavy makeup, jewelry (except for a wedding band, one small earring in each ear, wristwatch with a second hand), visible tattoos, and body piercings. Long hair must be tied back off the shoulders. Most faculty within schools of nursing strictly enforce the dress code, and students who deviate from the dress code or attempt to "jazz up" the uniform to make a personal statement run the risk of being dismissed from the clinical site. I remember during one of my clinical rotations the clinical instructor had to threaten to dismiss a student who refused to wear a bra. I know the student was not trying to be sexually provocative; however, her not wearing one had drawn the attention of hospital staff who brought their concerns to the clinical instructor. This was awkward for everyone—student, staff, and nursing instructor—involved and could have been avoided.

Sidebar 12-2

Do's and Don'ts for Getting the Most Out of the Clinical Experience

1. *Do not work the night before clinical.* There are students who work the night before coming to clinical. These students risk arriving at the clinical setting exhausted and incapable of safely caring for patients. Faculty often send exhausted and fatigued students home, and the students miss a clinical day. Students should arrange their schedule so that they are not working the night before the day of clinical. In fact, the night before clinical should be a time in which the student is preparing for clinical by reading, looking up drugs, obtaining a clinical assignment, and so on.
2. *Get a good night's sleep the night before clinical.* The evening before clinical is not the time to go out or do anything that will prevent you from showing up for clinical sharp and mentally ready to learn and safely care for patients.

3. *Eat before going to clinical.* Do not go to clinical on an empty stomach. Students who go to clinical on an empty stomach run the risk of having their blood sugar dropping, which can lead to fatigue and safety issues for both student and patients. Students who cannot eat first thing in the morning should bring something with them to eat later like a breakfast bar. Keep in mind that you may not have lunch until one or two in the afternoon, so bring a healthy snack and a bottle of water to keep in your bag to have in the late morning if needed. You may not be able to leave the clinical unit to go to the cafeteria and get a snack or a drink if the clinical day is busy, and it usually is.

4. *Don't just plan on arriving to clinical on time; show up early.* Clinical time is precious, and students should make every effort to show up to their clinical site early. The day before clinical students should have their uniform ready and their clinical equipment packed so they are not rushing around the day of clinical. Make sure that you are wearing the correct uniform of the school (see student handbook). This includes shoes, hair, etc. Heavy makeup, jewelry, and artificial nails are problematic. Students with visible tattoos on the arms and wrists may be asked to wear long sleeves. Stick to the student handbook, and avoid problems later on. There are faculty who send students home when they are not appropriately dressed and groomed for clinical, and they have the right to do so.

5. *Do what your current clinical instructor tells you to do.* All clinical instructors have a slightly different way of doing things, and students have to follow the directions of their current clinical instructor—not their previous clinical instructor.

6. *Be prepared and eager to learn.* Prior to the clinical experience the student should be prepared to give excellent nursing care to the assigned patient(s) (e.g., be familiar with diagnosis, medications, teaching plan, etc.). Moreover, students should be eager to learn as much as they can from the clinical instructor, nursing staff, and other healthcare providers at the clinical site. If you run into a problem on the clinical unit, go to your instructor *first*. He or she will then guide you in the correct resolution. Remember that you are a "guest" at the institution.

Jeanne Ruggiero, PhD, RN, APN-C
Assistant Professor, College of Nursing
Seton Hall University

Clinical Writing Assignments

The nursing care plan is the most common type of clinical writing assignment and is based upon the needs of a patient whom the student cared for in a specific clinical setting. For example, care plans you develop for your pediatric patients will be different from the care plans you develop for your medical–surgical patients. When I was in nursing school all students were required to complete nursing care plans. At that time most nursing educators believed that the student care plan was essential for nursing students to develop problem-solving skills, to apply the steps of the nursing process (i.e., assessment, nursing diagnosis, planning, implementation, and evaluation), to learn the skills of written and verbal communication, and to integrate theoretical knowledge to clinical practice (Potter & Perry, 2004). The nursing care plan was formatted so that each column represented a step in the nursing process. While many nursing educators still have students complete nursing care plans, a growing number of nursing educators have become critical of traditional nursing care plans (Mueller, Johnston, & Bligh, 2001, 2002) and have instituted such alternative forms of clinical writing assignments as concept mapping (Schuster, 2000). Whatever form of clinical writing assignment is required in your program, remember that these assignments are designed to enhance your critical thinking skills and clinical reasoning, so give yourself enough time to work on the assignment.

Sidebar 12-3

Tips for Care Plans

In most nursing programs students are required to develop care plans during clinical. While the care plan may not be due until the end of the clinical experience, it is in the best interest of students to start collecting clinical data early in the semester. Students should not wait until a week before the care plan is due to collect the clinical data they will need because there is no way to ensure that they will get a patient with enough information to write a care plan. For example, in the clinical days before the care plan is due, a student might end up getting a patient who is going to be in endoscopy all day or off the floor getting a test, and the student will not be able to interview and assess the patient and obtain enough data to write a care plan. If students start collecting clinical data early they will have a range of patients to choose from.

Jeanne Ruggiero, PhD, RN, APN-C
Assistant Professor, College of Nursing
Seton Hall University

The Clinical Day

Although a growing number of nursing programs are providing opportunities for students to perform clinical hours in subacute and community settings (e.g., Head Start centers, home care providers),[1] the focus of the discussion in this section is on clinical hours performed in acute care settings because most clinical hours during nursing school are performed in acute care settings such as medical–surgical units.

---

1. In some programs students spend a clinical day with their instructor in a simulation lab with pre-programmed scenarios, which allows students to practice their skills in a controlled environment and gives clinical faculty more time to evaluate the students' critical thinking abilities.

Preclinical Preparation

As discussed above, the clinical experience in most nursing programs entails 12 hours of clinical per week. Depending on a variety of factors (e.g., availability of clinical faculty, clinical sites), the 12 hours can be split over 2 days, 2 evenings, lumped into 1 day, or done on the weekend. In most nursing programs students are given clinical assignments prior to their clinical day. Thus, if your clinical day is Tuesday your clinical assignment will be made by your clinical instructor on Monday. If you are performing your clinical rotation in an acute care setting, such as a medical–surgical unit in a hospital, you are given the clinical assignment so that you can prepare yourself to provide care to the patient. For clinical experiences in acute settings, this preparation typically involves reviewing the patient's medical record to gather information such as the patient's admitting diagnosis, medications, and treatments. This review prepares the student to provide care for the patient, which may include administering the patient's medication, educating the patient about eating healthier, and discharge planning.

Preconference

On the scheduled clinical day, students meet with the clinical instructor and fellow students to discuss how they have prepared for the clinical day and exchange other pertinent clinical information prior to caring for patients. Typically, each student reviews his or her assignment and gives a thumbnail sketch of the patient and the diagnosis, medications, foley, oxygen, and other details. Depending on the number of students in the clinical and on how much feedback and instruction the clinical instructor provides during the preconference, these meetings can last anywhere from a few minutes to more than half an hour.

Clinical Time

Following the preconference, students begin their clinical day and over the next several hours start implementing their care plan. This includes receiving an update on the patient from the primary nurse, reviewing the medical records for updated information (e.g., laboratory studies, vital signs, and scheduled procedures), and introducing themselves to the patient. Another feature of many clinical experiences involves observations during the clinical day, and it is not uncommon for clinical instructors to arrange additional clinical experiences for students, such as observing surgery or spending the clinical day in the emergency department.

Sidebar 12-4

Medical Math

Prior to beginning their clinical experiences, most nursing programs require that students demonstrate they can perform the basic mathematical calculations they will need in the clinical setting such as calculating the intravenous rate, converting from kilograms to pounds, and checking medication dosages. Unfortunately, many students have difficulty in this area. Prior to taking the medical math portion of their nursing education, students should get the book and review all the basic mathematical operations they need to know that are covered in the introductory chapters. Most of this basic math is also discussed in other books such as those designed to help students prepare for the General Educational Development (GED) test. If you know basic arithmetic skills and mathematical skills (algebraic equations, ratios, percentages), the metric system and conversions to metric, you will have an easier time with medical math. Pay close attention to this; most schools consider an 80 or below a failure in a medical math test and, depending on school policies, you may have to repeat the course.

Jeanne Ruggiero, PhD, RN, APN-C
Assistant Professor, College of Nursing
Seton Hall University

Postconference

The last minutes (30–60 minutes) of each clinical day are spent in what is referred to as the postconference. The format for postconferences varies by program and clinical instructor; however, usually during this time students discuss matters such as interesting clinical situations, evaluation of their care plan, and problems that may have arisen. As with the preconference, students receive feedback, instruction, and encouragement from the clinical instructor.

Sidebar 12-5

Learn to Be a Colleague

I learned early in my career the importance of developing collegial relationships with my fellow nurses. In the hospital where I worked when I graduated from nursing school, I was the only BSN (Bachelor of Science in Nursing) graduate. Most of my nurse colleagues at that hospital were diploma school graduates who had received more preparation in the technical aspects of nursing as part of their nursing education than I had. I remember the first time I had to put in an NG tube (nasogastric tube), and I was nervous because I had only put in one NG tube during nursing school so I said to one of my colleagues who was a diploma grad—her name was Henrietta, but I liked to call her Hank—"Come on, Hank, you are going to watch me put in this NG tube."

Hank asked, "You've put in an NG tube before haven't you?"

I said, "Just once, which is why I want you to come and watch me." And this happened all the time in the first year or so that I worked there. However, there were other times that my colleagues would ask me for help especially when it related to tasks such as care plans. The BSN program that I graduated from, like most BSN programs, emphasized learning activities that promoted problem-solving skills rather than technical skills; thus, even as a new nurse, I was able to help my colleagues with such tasks as care plans that involved clinical decision making. After a few months of being there, a couple of my fellow nurses told me that they finally figured out how their training as diploma nurses differed from my training in a baccalaureate program. I told them I wasn't sure what they meant, and they told me that when we ask you nursing practice kinds of questions you know how to think it through, but at the same time you have no problem coming to us and consulting with us or asking for help when you have a question.

Successful nursing practice requires the ability to develop collegial relationships with nurses and other healthcare providers (e.g., physicians, social workers, physical therapists). Collegial relationships develop in health care when individuals share resources such as information and knowledge to improve the health of patients. Nursing students should practice working as colleagues, and the clinical conferences are a perfect time to implement this practice. Listen closely to what other students discuss in preclinical and postclinical meetings. Moreover, begin to practice the interpersonal and collegial roles you will assume as a nursing professional by asking questions of your peers and acting as a resource for your peers. Many students make the mistake of sitting passively through the clinical conferences and allowing the clinical instructor to ask all the questions and provide all of the answers.

Randolph Rasch, PhD, RN
Professor and Director of the Family Nurse Practitioner Specialty
Vanderbilt University School of Nursing

Nursing Clinicals and Stress

The few studies on the experiences of nursing students during the clinical portion of their nursing education indicate that for most nursing students, the challenges of clinical are more stressful than the challenges in the classroom. Why are nursing school clinicals so stressful? One reason may be that, in addition to the pressures of learning a substantial amount of material in a short amount of time, when nursing students begin performing nursing tasks in a healthcare setting, they have the additional pressures of making sure that they contribute to the promotion, maintenance, and restoration of the health of their patients (Wilson, 1994). These tasks are very different than discussing theoretical perspectives of caregiving in a classroom or providing care to a mannequin in the learning lab and can be extremely stressful.

Sidebar 12-6

Patients Need You to Be Confident

Most students are going to be anxious as they begin their clinical rotations. There is nothing wrong with feeling anxious, but it is important to remember that the patient is probably more nervous than you are and is looking for someone who knows what they are doing to help them ease their anxiety. You can be that someone if you project confidence. Here are some tips on how you can project confidence while you are feeling anxious:

1. *Be prepared before you enter the room.* Know everything that you can about the patient in terms of diagnosis and laboratory results before entering the room. Patients will not place their confidence in you if you do not have a handle on what is going on with them.
2. *Introduce yourself.* When you enter the patient's room speak clearly and confidently letting the patient know who you are (e.g., Hi, I am Charlie Hustle. I am a student nurse, and I will be here until 2 pm.)
3. *Let the patient know you have a plan.* Tell the patient what your plan for him or her is for the time you are there. If you are planning to give them a bed bath, administer medications, and provide discharge planning, let the patient know that.
4. *Ask the patient what they need.* Let the patient know that you are there to help them. For example, often patients are being seen by swarms of healthcare providers (e.g., physicians, medical students, social workers, etc.), and they have a lot of questions about their diagnosis and plan of care. You, in your role as a nursing student have the time and resources (e.g., knowledge) to help them make sense of what is going on.

Joy Atkins, MA, RN
Adjunct Instructor, Department of Nursing
Rutgers, The State University of New Jersey

In addition to the concerns relating to not being able to perform the tasks that they need to perform to care for patients (and to receive a passing grade in clinical), there are other concerns that contribute to the stress and anxiety of nursing students. Parkes (1985) conducted a qualitative study of first-year nursing students in Great Britain and found that these stressors could be categorized as follows:

1. Death of patients and issues of death and dying—For example, issues of death in the clinical setting evoke painful memories for the student.
2. Interpersonal difficulties with other nurses—This would include feeling unsupported and being treated inappropriately by nursing staff.
3. Interpersonal difficulties with patients such as uncooperative patients
4. Work overload, which includes being asked to carry out complex or unfamiliar tasks and being asked to do too much
5. Concerns about nursing care Examples include insensitivity toward patients or relatives and patients in severe care being left unattended.

Although Parkes' study is more than two decades old these stressors are still relevant today.

Sidebar 12-7

Make Patients Open to Your Care

To make a difference in the health of patients, nurses and other healthcare providers have to make patients open to the care they want to provide. Getting patients to become open to your care begins by gaining the confidence of your patients. One way to increase the chances of quickly gaining the confidence of your patient is to display self-confidence. This is not always easy when one is inexperienced as a nurse, but as the saying goes, "Fake it until you make it." When you walk into the patient's room, walk with your head up and walk with purpose. When you speak to the patient, speak clearly and make appropriate eye contact.

Elizabeth Ann Atkins, MA, RN
Clinical Director
Kennedy Health System

Handling the Stress of the Clinical Experience

As discussed in the section above, nursing students in the clinical have a great deal to worry about. Although anxiety has been shown to motivate action and may enhance performance and learning, high levels of anxiety can cause one to freeze up and can decrease learning (Kleehammer, Hart, & Keck, 1990). Provided in this section are some recommendations on how to avoid the levels of anxiety that can diminish learning and prevent one from getting the most out of the clinical experience in nursing school.

Sidebar 12-8

Red Flags to Report to the Clinical Instructor Immediately

Especially in the early clinical experiences, clinical instructors do not expect students to know how to manage the majority of clinical problems that may arise; however, clinical instructors do expect that students will report clinical red flags (discussed below) and report when there are discrepancies in the clinical report.

Clinical instructors are there to guide students and keep them out of potentially dangerous clinical situations; however, if students do not alert clinical instructors to what is going on with patients, then clinical instructors cannot do their job. Some red flags that students should report to clinical instructors immediately include: (1) low or high blood pressure (systolic < 110 or > 140 and diastolic < 60 or > 90); (2) heart rate greater than 100; and (3) abnormal breath sounds (e.g., wheeze, shortness of breath). Follow the guidelines of your clinical instructor or ask her or him for guidelines.

Jeanne Ruggiero, PhD, RN, APN-C
Assistant Professor, College of Nursing
Seton Hall University

Be Prepared

Of all the actions that you can take to reduce your anxiety around the clinical experience, the most important is to come to clinical prepared. As discussed, in most nursing programs you are given patient assignments by your clinical instructors at least 24 hours before clinical and you are then expected to do all that is needed so that you are prepared to provide care to the patients prior to coming to clinical. This preparation includes understanding the patient's diagnosis and being prepared to implement the appropriate nursing interventions (e.g., administering medications and treatments, providing education).[2] In most cases preparing for the patient assignment involves gathering research from a variety of sources (e.g., textbooks, journals); however, sometimes you may need to go an extra step. For example, if you were assigned a patient who was going to require urinary catheterization and you had only practiced that procedure

---

2. In addition to diminishing your learning by amplifying your anxiety, inadequate preparation may diminish your learning (and your grade) by leading to your dismissal from the clinical site. Many student handbooks of nursing programs warn students that failure to adequately prepare for clinical will result in dismissal from the clinical site. Many clinical instructors take this rule very seriously and, of course, you cannot get the most out of clinical if you are not there.

in a learning lab (on a mannequin), you might want to closely review the procedure in your textbook or return to the learning lab to practice. Remember that your learning as a nursing student is in your control because there is some evidence that the quality of your learning is influenced by the quality of your preparation (Windsor, 1987).

Remember That Most Students Feel Like an Impostor in the Beginning

Despite being prepared for the clinical experience, many nursing students are still plagued with feelings that they are impostors. The *impostor phenomenon* was a term first coined by Clance and Imes (1978) to describe an internal feeling of intellectual phoniness, chronic self-doubt regarding one's abilities, and fear that others will discover that one is a fraud. There is some empirical evidence that nursing students and other healthcare provider students are prone to such feelings and that this feeling contributes to psychological distress (Henning, Ey, & Shaw 1998). Moreover, anecdotal evidence suggests that many nursing students do feel like impostors as they begin their first clinical rotation. For example, I can still recall the feeling of being an impostor as I was about to begin my first clinical rotation in nursing school. I remember thinking, "I don't know enough yet, and it is only a matter of time before my clinical instructor figures it out." Many colleagues and students I have spoken with have also admitted to having similar feelings of self-doubt as they prepared to begin their clinicals in nursing school. An important step in handling the anxiety and distress that accompany feelings that you are an impostor is to work on replacing these illogical and inaccurate thoughts of being an impostor with more positive self-talk.

Use Positive Self-Talk

Self-talk or intrapersonal communication is the conversation that we carry on with ourselves throughout the day. This conversation can take a variety of forms. For example, it can be informative (e.g., I have a dentist appointment at 9 am today) or humorous (e.g., A horse walks into a bar and the bartender says, "Why the long face?"). Our interest is in the form of self-talk that has been termed *positive*. The use of positive self-talk has been linked to the reduction of anxiety (Weikle, 1993) and in improving performance (Goodhart, 1986) and, when used constructively, may contribute to you getting the most out of nursing school.

How does one use self-talk constructively? To begin using self-talk constructively you must recognize that your personal speech influences your thoughts, feelings, and behaviors. You then need to think about your internal dialogue and determine which of your internal conversations diminish anxiety and lead to a sense of well-being and which internal conversations heighten your psychological distress (Levine, 1991). Obviously, your goal is to increase the self-talk that improves the way you feel and decrease the self-talk that results in feelings of inadequacy and uncertainty. Because you are the sender and receiver when it comes to self-talk, one way to increase the positive self-talk is to send more positive self-talk to yourself. The positive self-talk that I refer to does not include narcissistic self-love talk (e.g., I am God's gift to nursing) or grandiose delusions (e.g., I can heal with my voice). I refer to talk that is constructive, grounded in reality, and contributes to higher levels of functioning.

Here are some examples of how you can use self-talk to your advantage in the clinical setting:

1. Instead of telling yourself you are an impostor, tell yourself that every health-care provider was a student at one time and that many of them also felt like impostors.
2. Instead of talking to yourself about all of the things you do not know (e.g., how to intubate, read an X-ray), talk to yourself about all the things that you do know (e.g., how to perform CPR, educate patients about their medications).
3. Tell yourself that you have been preparing for clinical since you began nursing school and that you have done your best to prepare for this clinical day.
4. Instead of talking to yourself about how anxious you feel about providing care, talk to yourself about how fortunate you are to be in the position to provide nursing care to another human being—I am going to help someone feel better today!
5. Tell yourself that you are not alone but part of a healthcare team that includes your nursing instructor and the staff of the clinical setting (e.g., nursing staff, medical staff).

Pick Your Battles

A number of stressors contribute to the anxiety and psychological distress of nursing students during clinical rotations. Developing positive ways to cope with these stressors (versus maladaptive ways like smoking, drinking, and use of medication) is important for getting the most out of nursing school and for your future in the nursing profession. Latack (1986) found that individuals who developed positive ways to cope with stressors in the workplace were less likely to report job-related anxiety, dissatisfaction, and burnout. Although a great deal of research has been conducted regarding coping with workplace stressors, a study conducted by Parkes (1990) on a sample of trainee teachers is especially relevant to reducing the anxiety and psychological distress that may occur during the clinical experience. She found that participants who scored high on measures of suppression (e.g., restraint, compromise, and continuing with immediate activities regardless of difficulties) were less stressed than their counterparts with lower scores on these measures. This finding, which is consistent with the findings from other studies that have looked at the role of suppression as a coping mechanism, suggests that you help yourself out by being judicious in what you express. Just because you feel something does not mean you always have to express it. For example, your clinical instructor may have a preference in how things are documented that goes against what you learned in class or a previous clinical, and your instructor may have directed you and your classmates to follow her preference. While it is hard to bite your tongue when you feel you want to say something, it may be to your advantage to hold back.

Sidebar 12-9

Set Personal Objectives and Share Your Clinical Goals with Nursing Instructor

Students need to be proactive to get the most out of the clinical experiences. As a nursing student there were a number of experiences that I missed because I was not proactive in seeking out clinical experiences. One way for students to get the most out of the clinical experiences is to develop personal learning goals for each clinical experience that they then share with their clinical instructor. This is not to say that clinical instructors can always satisfy these requests, but clinical instructors want students to have varied clinical experiences and being aware of what students have seen clinically will help instructors achieve this aim. The need to vary clinical experiences becomes especially true during later clinicals as students get more clinical experiences under their belt and they may find that they are seeing patients with similar diagnoses and performing a limited range of procedures. For example, a student may have had the opportunity to do numerous wound dressings but never performed tracheotomy care. The student should let the clinical instructor know where there are gaps in clinical experiences.

Cynthia Ayres, PhD, RN
Assistant Professor, College of Nursing
Rutgers, The State University of New Jersey

Work with Your Classmates

I am not certain but I would imagine that there are some professions in which being a team player is not an asset. I am certain that nursing is not one of those professions, and for nurses the importance of working as part of a team becomes evident during nursing school clinicals. There is evidence that nursing students who can support and be supported by their classmates will get more out of clinical than their peers who attempt to go solo. Nursing school classmates are a valuable resource, and students who treat the clinical experience as a competition and their classmates as competitors not only increase their stress level unnecessarily, but they also deny themselves access to this resource. Campbell, Larrivee, Field, Day, and Reutter (1994) found that nursing students do better in clinical when they support each other's learning, provide emotional support, and assist each other with clinical tasks. The clinical experiences are challenging emotionally, physically, and intellectually; so if you see a classmate who looks like he or she needs something you can offer, do not hesitate to give it.

Don't Try to Fly Under the Radar During Clinical

One source of anxiety for many students stems from the awareness that they are being evaluated. Students want to look good in their roles as student nurses, and many worry that the clinical nursing instructor will observe them making some sort of blunder (e.g., medication error, not knowing the answer to a patient's question) that makes them look like they do not know what they are doing (Kleehammer et al., 1990; Wilson, 1994). Some students handle the concern that they will be evaluated poorly by trying to *fly under the radar,* thereby avoiding the clinical instructor during the clinical day. This approach heightens anxiety and diminishes learning because the student spends the clinical experience worried about avoiding the clinical instructor rather than focusing on what he or she ought to be learning during the clinical experience. Moreover, this approach of avoiding the clinical instructor contributes to a sense that the clinical instructor is the enemy or an adversary. Developing an adversarial dynamic with the clinical instructor diminishes learning because there is some evidence to suggest that the nursing student learns more from the clinical instructors than teachers in the classroom (Campbell et al., 1994) and that students who have a good relationship with clinical instructors learn more (Campbell et al., 1994; Griffith & Bakanauskas, 1983; Kleehammer et al., 1990). You can decrease your anxiety and take an active role in shaping your learning by developing an open and nonadversarial relationship with the clinical instructor. It is unlikely that you are going to become best buddies with your clinical instructor, but your clinical instructor can become an ally in your learning if you put in the effort. For example, there is nothing wrong with admitting to the clinical instructor that you are nervous about putting in a Foley catheter and asking the clinical instructor for tips that may not have been discussed in your textbook or that you may have not picked up in the learning lab. Remember that most clinical instructors have become educators because they like to teach and they care about the nursing profession.

Just Keep Showing Up

The first clinical day of the first clinical experience is a terrifying and anxiety-inducing experience for most nursing students; however, one important point to remember about the clinical experiences of nursing school is, if you keep showing up, it is probably going to get better. In fact most studies of nursing students suggest that the first clinical experiences produced the highest levels of anxiety (Jones & Johnston, 1997). With time, students start to feel more at ease with clinical and by the end of their nursing school careers, many students enjoy clinical. Windsor (1987) interviewed nursing students and found that nursing students go through three distinct learning stages during their clinical rotations. In the first stage, where anxiety was highest, students focused on performing nursing tasks. In the second stage, students sought to identify the roles of nurses. And in the third stage, students no longer were so concerned about performing nursing tasks and were interested in more autonomy.

Sidebar 12-10

What Is an Accu-Chek?

I like teaching clinical, and one of my most memorable experiences in teaching occurred while I was a medical–surgical clinical instructor. I had a class of students who, for the most part, were well-prepared and making good progress in their ability to provide care for patients; however, I realized that one student in the class, I'll call him Justin, seemed to lag behind his peers. The reason for Justin's slower rate of development as compared to his peers did not have to do with a lack of preparation or that he was not as smart as his peers; in fact, Justin had strong grades in his theory courses. I believe the difference in Justin's clinical progress could be explained by two factors. First, he lacked common sense, which I have learned is a not uncommon problem. Second, and perhaps more

continues

problematic, was that Justin was reluctant to take responsibility for the care that he provided and, instead, he would spend a great deal of his clinical time seeking me out to ask questions that he could find an answer to on his own (e.g., "Where is the blood pressure cuff?") or request that I assist him with tasks that he should have been able to handle on his own by that point in his nursing school career (e.g., "Could you help me record the urine output for this patient?").

I realized that I was spending a disproportionate amount of time answering his questions and overseeing his care, which was not fair to his classmates. The straw that broke the camel's back came one day when he asked me, "What is an Accu-Chek?" holding the plastic device, which was about the size of a garage door opener. As a 3rd-year nursing student, he had learned about Accu-Cheks, which are blood glucose monitoring systems for patients with diabetes, in his theory courses, clinical courses, and clinical labs. Frustrated, I told him to go ask one of his peers in the class. When he returned 10 minutes later, I noticed that three of his male peers were trailing behind him with mischievous smiles. I asked Justin if he had found out what an Accu-Chek was and he informed me he had. "You put the Accu-Chek strip in a woman's vagina to determine whether she is pregnant," he said confidently. His friends in the class burst into laughter. I am not sure it was the most professional thing to do, but I also found myself laughing heartily as I pictured Justin going into the room of a female patient with diabetes and telling her that he was going to put the Accu-Chek probe into her vagina to see if she was pregnant.

Kathy Abel, MSN, RN
Adjunct Lecturer, College of Nursing
Rutgers, The State University of New Jersey

References

Campbell, I. E., Larrivee, L., Field, P. A., Day, R. A., & Reutter, L. (1994). Learning to nurse in the clinical setting. *Journal of Advanced Nursing, 20,* 1125–1131.

Clance, P. R., & Imes, S. A. (1978). The impostor phenomenon in high-achieving women: Dynamics and therapeutic intervention. *Psychotherapy: Theory, Research and Practice, 15,* 241–247.

Goodhart, D. E. (1986). The effects of positive and negative thinking on performance in an achievement situation. *Journal of Personality and Social Psychology, 51,* 117–124.

Griffith, J. W., & Bakanauskas, A. J. (1983). Student-instructor relationships in nursing education. *Journal of Nursing Education, 22*(3), 104–107.

Hedderwick, S., McNeil, S., Lyons, M., & Kauffman, C. (2000). Pathogenic organisms associated with artificial fingernails worn by healthcare workers. *Infection Control and Hospital Epidemiology, 21,* 8.

Henning, K., Ey, S., & Shaw, D. (1998). Perfectionism, the impostor phenomenon, and psychological adjustment in medical, dental, nursing, and pharmacy students. *Medical Education, 32,* 456–464.

Jones, M. C., & Johnston, D. W. (1997). Distress, stress and coping in first-year student nurses. *Journal of Advanced Nursing, 26,* 475–482.

Kleehammer, K., Hart, A. L., & Keck, J. F. (1990). Nursing students' perceptions of anxiety-producing situations in the clinical setting. *Journal of Nursing Education, 29,* 183–187.

Latack, J. C. (1986). Coping with job stress. *Journal of Applied Psychology, 71,* 377–385.

Leighow, S. R. (1996). Backrubs vs. Bach: Nursing and the entry into practice debate, 1946–1986. *Nursing History Review, 4,* 3–18.

Levine, B. H. (1991). *Your body believes every word you say: The language of the body/mind connection.* Boulder Creek: Asian.

Mangum, S., Garrison, C., Lind, C., & Hilton, H. G. (1997). First impressions of the nurse and nursing care. *Journal of Nursing Care Quality, 11*(5), 39–47.

Mangum, S., Garrison, C., Lind, C., Thackeray, R., & Wyatt, M. (1991). Perceptions of nurses' uniforms. *Image—the Journal of Nursing Scholarship, 23*(2), 127–130.

McNeil, S., Foster, C., Hedderwick, S., & Kauffman, C. (2001). Effect of hand cleaning with antimicrobial soap or alcohol-based gel on microbial colonization of artificial fingernails worn by healthcare workers. *Clinical Infections Disease, 32,* 367–372.

Moolenaar, R. L., Crutcher, J. M., San Joaquin, V. H., Sewell, L. V., Hutwagner, L. C., Carson, L. A., et al. (2000). A prolonged outbreak of pseudomonas aeruginosa in a neonatal intensive care unit: Did staff fingernails play a role in disease transmission? *Infection Control and Hospital Epidemiology: The Official Journal of the Society of Hospital Epidemiologists of America, 21,* 80–85.

Mueller, A., Johnston, M., & Bligh, D. (2001). Mind-mapped care plans: A remarkable alternative to traditional nursing care plans. *Nurse Educator, 26,* 75–80.

Mueller, A., Johnston, M., & Bligh, D. (2002). Viewpoint: Joining mind mapping and care planning to enhance student critical thinking and achieve holistic nursing care. *Nursing Diagnosis, 13,* 24–27.

Parkes, K. (1990). Coping, negative affectivity, and the work environment: Addictive and interactive predictors of mental health. *Journal of Applied Psychology, 75,* 399–409.

Parkes, K. R. (1985). Stressful episodes reported by first-year student nurses: A descriptive account. *Social Science Medicine, 20,* 945–953.

Potter, P. A., & Perry, A. G. (2004). *Fundamentals of nursing.* Philadelphia: Mosby.

Schuster, P. M. (2000). Concept mapping: Reducing clinical care plan paperwork and increasing learning. *Nurse Educator, 25,* 76–81.

Tanner, C. A. (2006). The next transformation: Clinical education. *Journal of Nursing Education, 45,* 99–100.

Weikle, J. E. (1993). Self-talk and health. *ERIC Digest.* Retrieved August 10, 2007, from http://www.indiana.edu/~reading/ieo/digests/d84.html

Wilson, M. E. (1994). Nursing student perspective of learning in a clinical setting. *Journal of Nursing Education, 33,* 81–86.

Windsor, A. (1987). Nursing students' perceptions of clinical experience. *Journal of Nursing Education, 26,* 150–154.

THIRTEEN

Managing Your Time During Nursing School

Getting the most out of nursing school requires that you prioritize your nursing school education. While most researchers agree that intellectual and educational achievements require time and perseverance, few researchers have investigated the role of time management on educational achievement (Britton & Tesser, 1991). Britton and Tesser conducted one of the few studies looking at the relation of time management to academic achievement and they found that after controlling for SAT scores, there was a significant association between one's ability to manage time effectively during freshman year and cumulative GPA four years later. Individuals vary in the extent to which they are effective at managing their time; however, as with other skills (e.g., playing the piano, knitting), time management skills can be developed. Discussed in this section are some of the characteristics of effective time managers and tips for improving your ability to manage time in school and your daily life.

Sidebar 13-1

Nursing Students Who Are Parents: Reframe the Experience

I have taught quite a few students who are also parents, and I have heard their frustrations. Especially for women, because of the culture and society we live in, many feel extremely guilty about going to clinical and dropping their child off at the babysitter or day care when the child has the sniffles or just not spending the same amount of time with their child as other parents because of all the work they have to do in nursing school. While I understand these frustrations, I think it is important for students who are also parents and already committed to pursuing a nursing education to "flip" or reframe the nursing school experience. I try to get them to consider the extent to which they are a role model for their children as they pursue their education, prioritize, and make sacrifices to accomplish their goal of becoming a nurse. There is not much use in thinking,: "I am a bad parent because I am not spending quality time with my child"; it does nothing for the student or their child. It is better to reframe the experience of nursing school so that the student realizes they are making a short-term sacrifice that will benefit them and their child in the long term. And this "reframing" is also what we as nurses need to be able to help patients with also. We all have expectations and we have reality. Many times the two do not match, and when that happens there is no use banging one's head against the wall.

Nanette Sulik, MSN, RN
Clinical Instructor, Department of Nursing
Rutgers, The State University of New Jersey

Make a List of the Things That You Have to Do Each Day

To most effectively manage time it is important to first determine what has to be done in the time you have. One of the most effective ways to do this is to take the time to compile a list (a to-do list) of the tasks that need to be completed each day. Some people use high-tech methods to compile their lists (e.g., personal data assistants [PDAs]) while others keep the list through various low-tech means (e.g., old envelopes). How one compiles the list is unimportant; what matters is that you physically document what needs to be done and you refer to the list throughout the day. Why is the list such a valuable time management tool? Many people find that they procrastinate less and feel better when they have a physical reminder of what has to be done (Bond & Feathern, 1988). In addition, keeping a list makes it less likely that you will forget the minor tasks that often slip through the cracks. Finally, it provides a psychic charge to cross tasks off your list and reduces the psychic burden of wondering what you forgot to do.

Planning

How does one go about compiling a list? Making a list begins by thinking and planning what needs to be done in the short term (e.g., in the next 24 hours) and what should be completed in the long term (in the next few weeks or by the end of the semester). As a student you will usually know what you will have to complete by the end of the semester (e.g., one research paper, two case studies, two midterms) and when these assignments are due. You should definitely know what you have to work with in terms of time resources. If you allot at least 8 hours per day to sleep (and most of the research on sleep says that most of us function better if we do), there are 112 waking hours in a week. Of course, all of your waking time will not be devoted to completing your work in nursing school: most students have other activities they do because they want to (e.g., community service, socializing with friends and family) or because they have to (e.g., work, child care). However, based on the due dates of assignments, you can begin making rough estimates of how much time you should need to complete assignments.

For example, if you have a paper due on April 15, you want to decide on a date to have completed each step of the assignment (e.g., April 13: final draft due; April 10: rough draft due; April 7: complete research; April 1: select topic). In this way you do not end up scrambling on April 14 to write a paper that is due the next day. This also allows for mechanical problems (e.g., faulty printer, loss of electricity) that you cannot control.

Break It Down

Some students may feel a sense of anxiety after determining what tasks have to be completed during a semester and wonder "How will I get this all done?" In contrast, other students may look at what has to be done during the semester and think, "No problem, I have plenty of time." Developing a daily list will help those prone to anxiety and those prone to procrastination; however, each of these individuals has to spend some time breaking the tasks down to size. For example, a clinical research paper may be one of the assignments due at the end of the semester; however, as discussed in Chapter 10, that is not a task one can put on a daily list: it is not going to be completed in one day. Alternatively, there are components of the clinical research paper that one could probably complete in one day such as *develop an outline for the paper* in one day and in the next day one might be able to *start conducting online research*. In sum, one key to making the list an effective time management tool lies in the process of "breaking down" tasks to meaningful parts.

Setting Priorities

Your final consideration in keeping a daily list involves determining which tasks are most pressing and which ones can wait for tomorrow, next week, next month, or never. Which tasks take priority will depend on a number of factors (e.g., academic strengths, outside commitments). What is most important is that you figure out what has to be done right now and do that first.

Sidebar 13-2

Write a Letter to Your Family

In our program, like many other baccalaureate programs, junior year marks the point at which the demands of nursing school skyrocket, and it becomes difficult to maintain many of one's social and familial relationships. At the beginning of junior year I suggest to students that they write letters to the members of their family letting them know that they will not be around during the semester, but they will be home for holidays and semester breaks. For example, students who are part of families that have a tradition of eating Sunday dinner together need to explain to their family that they will not be able to attend every Sunday dinner during the semester because they need to study. While family members are typically disappointed to learn that they will see less of you during nursing school, as long as your family knows in advance that you are not rejecting them and that you will return to the routine after you complete your nursing studies, they are usually accepting.

However, students who have a "significant other" in their lives need to plan time to focus on that person. All relationships need to be nurtured, but this one needs special attention. Some successful students deliberately plan to close their books on Saturday night each week and go out with their special person. It might only involve a trip to the mall or the local coffee shop, but it is uninterrupted time for only that person. The plan communicates love and caring. Not to arrange this time suggests that this person is not important, and the student risks losing this person.

Jane Kurz, PhD, RN
Associate Professor, Department of Nursing
Temple University

Nursing School and Work

I have taught many students who have tried to work full- or part-time jobs while in nursing school. Too frequently, these students become deprived of sleep, then they get sick, and then they fall behind because they are not doing their work. I think what students need to realize more than anything else is that everything they do has consequences. Just as nursing students learn that everything they do in the clinical setting has consequences for patients, everything students do in their personal lives has consequences for them.

Nanette Sulik, MSN, RN
Clinical Instructor, Department of Nursing
Rutgers, The State University of New Jersey

Time Attitude

In addition to keeping a daily to-do list, higher-achieving students differ from lower-achieving students in their attitudes toward time management. Britton and Tesser (1991) found that higher-achieving students were more likely than lower-achieving students to avoid spending time on tasks that interfered with academic achievement. Higher-achieving students had a greater sense of control over time than their lower-achieving counterparts. Discussed below are some suggestions for adjusting your attitude toward time. In addition, a time management tool is provided in Appendix 13-A that will assist you in figuring out how you are spending your time and identify areas where you might be able to conserve time.

Protect Your Time

Time is a commodity, and like everyone else you have 24 hours to spend a day. While all of that time cannot (and should not) be spent on school, it is important that you do not allow your time to be wasted. It is amazing how much time can be consumed in activities that add nothing to your life. Develop the attitude that you are going to spend your time wisely. This might include the following:

- Grocery shop during off-peak hours (between 10 am and 4 pm) to avoid standing in line.
- Screen your phone calls, especially when the phone call is from an unknown number or during your time to study. If the call is important, the caller will leave a message.
- Opt not to become a pet owner or start a new hobby during nursing school.
- Keep note cards, a study book, or one of your textbooks with you when you leave the house so that if you get stuck in traffic or in a waiting room you can use the time to study.
- Pay your bills online.
- Stay away from the television. It will steal your time and give you little in return. The computer and cell phone can also steal time (e.g., Facebook, instant messaging, e-mailing, text messaging, watching videos on YouTube, and taking and sending pictures). Shut off your cell phone and resist the urge to check e-mail frequently.
- Set aside time in your calendar to study, the way you would make an appointment. Tell friends and family that you will be studying or writing during that time and to please not call you unless there is an emergency.

Wear a Watch

You might not like the feel or the look of a watch on your wrist, but try to get over the dislike and start wearing a watch. Time is a commodity and wearing a watch will give you a constant reminder of how you are spending your time. Moreover, you are going to need a watch that has a second hand in clinical to assess heart rate and respirations. Most cell phones have alarms that can be set as reminders.

Organize Work Habits

The third and final difference in time management practices that Britton and Tesser (1991) found between high- and low-achieving students was in how they organized their work habits to optimize their efficiency. For example, the higher-achieving students were less likely than lower-achieving students to report that they tried to split their attention between tasks (multitasking). This finding is consonant with findings from a growing number of studies that show that multitasking decreases productivity[1] (Gopher, Armony, & Greenspan, 2000; Yeung & Monsell, 2003).

In addition to remaining focused on tasks, higher-achieving students were more likely than their counterparts to report that they regularly reviewed their notes throughout the semester rather than cramming review of notes for the exam. Discussed below are some suggestions for organizing your work habits to optimize your study time.

Although there are no shortcuts to learning what you need to know as a nurse and you will have to work hard to learn the material and complete your assignments, your goal is to optimize your studying time so that you get the most out of every minute you spend studying. An integral step in making the most of your study time is to figure out what time of the day you are best able to study. There is some evidence to suggest that variations exist between individuals (morning types versus evening types) in when they reach their peak performance (Natale & Lorenzetti, 1997). Determine what time of day you seem to get the most out of your time studying, and use that time to study. In addition, figure out the study environment that works best for you. Some students study best in solitude and complete quiet, while others need some background noise. If you are constantly surrounded by noise, invest in a pair of inexpensive soft earplugs (available at any drugstore). A white noise machine, or a machine that provides a variety of nature sounds, can help drown out distracting noises.

Tips to Optimize Time Efficiency

Below are some other strategies that you may find useful to optimize your time:

1. **Plan to plan**—Making room in your day to plan the tasks that you hope to complete increases your sense of control, as well as your sense of accomplishment when you do complete tasks.
2. **Do not multitask**—Do not try to split your focus between tasks. There is evidence to suggest that your effectiveness decreases when you switch between tasks (Rubinstein, Meyer, & Evans, 2001). Complete one task, or as much of it as you can, before moving on to the next.

---

1. Meyer and Kieras (1997) found that even brief mental blocks created by shifting between tasks can cost as much as 40% of an individual's productivity.

3. **Prioritize your tasks**—All tasks are not equal. Decide what has to be done sooner rather than later and work on that first. For example, studying for the quiz you will have tomorrow morning should take priority over working on your care plan that is not due for a week.

4. **Just say no**—Consider your goals and schedule before agreeing to take on additional work. For example, if you are a parent of a school-aged child, nursing school is not the time to take on a Parent-Teacher Association (PTA) position.

5. **Do it right the first time**—In the long run it takes more time to correct errors than it does to do the work correctly the first time. Spend the extra time it takes to get it right. For example, when you find a reference that you want to use in a paper, accurately record the information that you will need to cite the reference (e.g., author's name, journal name, volume number) at the time you find the reference rather than having to go back and find that information at a later date.

6. **Break large, time-consuming tasks into smaller tasks**—Whenever a task seems overwhelming, think about how you can break the task down into smaller tasks.

7. **Practice the 10-minute rule**—Work on a dreaded task for 10 minutes each day. Once you get started, you may find you can finish it. For example, if you have a strong dislike for writing nursing care plans, start your study time with that task.

8. **Promote and maintain your own health**—Reduce the amount of time you spend out of action due to illness by getting adequate sleep and rest, making time for exercise (you can fit exercise into your day by getting in the habit of walking as much as possible and taking the stairs rather than the elevator), washing your hands (carry a small bottle of hand sanitizer for times when you are away from a sink), and eating a balanced and nutritious diet. Eat foods that are high in protein and low in refined sugar and carbohydrates. Sugar and refined carbohydrates may cause "highs" and "crashes." Include fruits and vegetables in all of your meals. Do not skip meals. Stay hydrated by drinking water or other beverages throughout the day. Even mild dehydration can lead to fatigue. Avoid beverages with heavy sugar content and caffeine. Read labels—even juice can be loaded with sweeteners.

9. **Be careful with the caffeine**—Avoid consuming too many caffeinated beverages. In excessive amounts, the temporary "highs" they provide often end in fatigue or a "crash" later. Moreover, these beverages may disrupt your sleep and make you feel jittery. A jittery, anxiety-ridden mind is not capable of

careful reasoning and focus. Heavy caffeine intake can also reduce attention span. Remember that no amount of caffeine can effectively keep you awake and functional if you are sleep deprived.

10. **Give yourself small rewards for task completion**—Find ways to reward yourself for completing tasks on your list and for not goofing off. Small rewards might include a 20-minute phone call to a loved one or 20 minutes of listening to music.

Sidebar 13-3

Working Students: 20-Hour Rule

Earning a degree in nursing school requires more of a time commitment than other degrees. We have found in our nursing program, and this is supported by the literature, that 20 hours seems to be the tipping point in terms of *maximum* number of hours that students can work and balance the demands of nursing school. Students who work more than 20 hours have difficulty in maintaining that balance and, in turn, that increases their likelihood of failing courses.

Jane Kurz, PhD, RN
Associate Professor, Department of Nursing
Temple University

Real-World Snapshot 13-2

Students with Children: Finding Time to Study

Success in nursing school requires blocks of uninterrupted time. Unfortunately, many students with young children often have trouble creating blocks of time that are sufficiently large enough to study or complete assignments in nursing school. One piece of advice I give to students with young children is to get the services of a babysitter as often as possible and to use that time to study or complete assignments without the demands of child care. Even if the student does not physically leave their home to study during this time, it is important for the student to be able to leave mentally and emotionally and focus on studying.

Jane Kurz, PhD, RN
Associate Professor, Department of Nursing
Temple University

References

Bond, M. J., & Feathern, N. T. (1988). Some correlates of structure and purpose in the use of time. *Journal of Personality and Social Psychology, 55,* 321–329.

Britton, B. K., & Tesser, A. (1991). Effects of time-management practices on college grades. *Journal of Educational Psychology, 83,* 405–410.

Gopher, D., Armony, L., & Greenspan, Y. (2000). Switching tasks and attention policies. *Journal of Experimental Psychology: General, 129,* 308–329.

Meyer, D. E., & Kieras, D. E. (1997). A computational theory of executive cognitive processes and multiple-task performance: Part 2. Accounts of psychological refractory-period phenomena. *Psychological Review, 104,* 749–791.

Natale, V., & Lorenzetti, R. (1997). Influences of morningness-eveningness and time of day on narrative comprehension. *Personality and Individual Differences, 23,* 685–690.

Rubinstein, J. S., Meyer, D. E., & Evans, J. E. (2001). Executive control of cognitive processes in task switching. *Journal of Experimental Psychology: Human Perception and Performance, 27*(4), 763–797.

Yeung, N., & Monsell, S. (2003). Switching between tasks of unequal familiarity: The role of stimulus-attribute and response-set selection. *Journal of Experimental Psychology: Human Perception and Performance, 29*(2), 455–469.

APPENDIX 13-A

Time Management Exercise: Are You Giving Yourself Enough Time to Get the Most out of Nursing School?

1. Fill out the schedule below for a typical week during the semester.

	Mon	Tues	Wed	Thurs	Fri	Sat	Sun
6:00 am							
7:00 am							
8:00 am							
9:00 am							
10:00 am							
11:00 am							
12:00 pm							
1:00 pm							
2:00 pm							
3:00 pm							
4:00 pm							
5:00 pm							
6:00 pm							
7:00 pm							
8:00 pm							
9:00 pm							
10:00 pm							
11:00 pm							

2. Use the schedule in Step 1 to determine how much time you spend in the activities listed below.

    A. School/Academic

        a. Commuting time   _____

        b. Class time   _____

        c. Clinical time   _____

        d. Studying[1]   _____

        e. Clinical preparation time[2]   _____

    B. Employment

        a. Commuting time   _____

        b. Weekly hours spent at work   _____

    C. Home/family/friends

        a. Child/elder care   _____

        b. Cooking/cleaning/shopping, etc. _____

        c. Socializing (going out, chatting) _____

    D. Personal

        a. Sleep   _____

        b. Eating   _____

        c. Hygiene   _____

        d. Exercise   _____

        e. "Me time" (e.g., hobbies, leisure) _____

        f. Religious/spiritual   _____

        g. Community service   _____

3. Total A through D and subtract from 168 (number of hours per week).

4. Now ask yourself the following questions to determine if you are giving yourself enough time to get the most out of nursing school:

    • Have I created enough time to study and prepare for clinical?

    • Is it possible to re-allocate my time so that I can focus on my nursing education?

    • Am I putting too much time into unprofitable activities?

---

1. Allocate 2 hours of studying time for each hour of class time.
2. Allocate 2 hours of clinical preparation time per 6 hours of clinical.

FOURTEEN

How to Take a Test in Nursing School

In nursing school most students will take all sorts of tests: quizzes, midterms, and final exams. For professors and the institution, tests provide a way to determine whether students have mastered the material they need to know. For students, tests are an opportunity to determine whether they are getting the most they can out of their nursing school education. If you score well on your exam it is likely you are making the most of your nursing school experience. If you do not score well, it may be you are having difficulty managing the demands of coursework in nursing school, you do not know how to take tests, or a combination of the two problems. In the previous chapters, discussion was provided on how to make the most out of your time in nursing school. In this chapter the focus will be on improving your ability to take the kinds of tests you are likely to encounter in nursing school.

Preparation

In Chapter 7 the importance of attending class, reading actively, and taking notes was discussed. You know that by approaching these activities strategically and systematically you learn more than if you just go through the motions. The same applies for preparing for tests: if you are just going through the motions you are unlikely to do your best. Your strategy for test preparation begins during the first week of the semester. This strategy involves not only reading the assigned material actively and taking lecture notes, but spending at least 10 minutes every week reviewing the notes that you have taken in your lecture notes and the reading. Pauk (1984) estimates that these periodic reviews will quadruple the amount of material you will be able to retain. The information you retain forms the foundation of your test preparation.

Sidebar 14-1

Look for the Intersections or Areas of Overlap

In figuring out what to study, students should look at their notes, the notes given from the professor, and the reading. Information or concepts that appear in the notes, class notes, and reading are probably important, and students should make a point of gaining a good understanding of this information.

Cynthia Ayres, PhD, RN
Assistant Professor, College of Nursing
Rutgers, The State University of New Jersey

Sidebar 14-2

Preparing for Nursing Exams

Most students have to adjust to taking nursing school exams as they are different from exams they have taken in other courses. Many of these students complain that there were two choices that seemed correct. Here are recommendations we have given to students to help them prepare for nursing exams:

- Don't wait until the day before the exam to begin studying—Many students have found cramming to be a successful strategy in studying for exams in nonnursing courses; however, we have found that students who are successful in taking nursing exams began studying for short periods of time well in advance of the nursing exam.
- Memorizing is not enough—Although there is some information that nursing students will probably have to memorize for their exams (e.g., 5 cc = 1 tsp.), most nursing exams reward students who are able to retain information and apply it using the nursing process.
- Look at the objectives on your course syllabi—In preparing for nursing exams students should refer frequently to the course objectives on the course syllabi. We advise students to see if they can answer the objectives in their own words and develop questions from the objectives on the course syllabi. This approach helps students to know the information that is important in that course but also forces students to think about applying that information.

• Do practice test questions—Another way to develop the ability to apply the information is through practice test questions. These questions can be found in NCLEX preparation books, nursing textbooks, and on the Internet. To get the most benefit out of practicing test questions, students should seek to understand the rationale for the correct and incorrect answers working individually or through group discussions.

Carol Carofiglio, PhD, RN
Nursing Faculty
Helene Fuld School of Nursing In Camden County

Sidebar 14-3

Tips for Studying for an Exam

• If the professor takes the time to provide a blueprint of the test, use it to guide your studying.
• Start studying at least a week before the exam is given. Cramming the night before is not going to get you where you want to be. You will be fatigued and very anxious. An anxious and fatigued mind cannot think critically and can lead the student to select wrong answers.
• Practice test questions and focus on the rationales. Go over your class notes, and look for those areas that intersect with the reading and the blueprint.
• Do not spend all of your study time memorizing information and facts. The tests that students will take in nursing are geared to test how well students apply the information. Plan time to study information and time to do test questions and read case studies in the textbook. Study the information *and* how to apply the information.
• If you are working during nursing school, schedule your vacation time so that it coincides with the times during the semester that you will need more time to study (e.g., midsemester and final exam week). Plan well in advance so your employer is more likely to honor your requests.
• If a test review is offered, make sure that you go to it. If a posttest review is offered, make sure that you go to it and see what test questions you got wrong and, more importantly, the kinds of test questions that you got wrong and *why*. Make sure that you focus on improving in the areas that you are weakest for the next test. You may need to change your studying habits. Ask your professor for help in this area. Standardized testing is administered by most nursing schools at various times in the student's nursing education. Results are compiled by the testing company to analyze each student's performance. Students receive individualized reports regarding their areas of strength and weakness. For example, a student report from a medical-surgical exam may indicate a weakness in understanding of fluid and electrolyte balance. Pay attention to these recommendations.

Jeanne Ruggiero, PhD, RN, APN-C
Assistant Professor, College of Nursing
Seton Hall University

Recitation

Most of us have also had an experience in which, while we wanted to retain information, we were not able to move it from our short-term memory to our long-term memory. This happens to me when I am driving and I stop to ask for directions. No sooner do I get back in the car than I have forgotten whether I am supposed to turn right or left at the second light. One important process that can be improved to retain information is known as recitation. As was discussed briefly in Chapter 7 (see discussion of SQ3R), recitation involves reciting the concepts that you want to remember. Most of us have had some learning experience that was enhanced by recitation. For example, many children learn the alphabet through song. This process improves the likelihood that you will transfer information from your short-term memory to your long-term memory.

In his book on studying in college, Pauk (1984) offers three good reasons for why recitation works:

1. Recitation lets you know how you are doing. A correct recitation is an immediate reward that helps to keep motivation high. An incorrect recitation is punishment that motivates a student to avoid future punishment by studying harder.
2. Recitation strengthens the original memory trace, because your mind must actively think about the new material.
3. The physical activity of thinking, pronouncing, and even hearing your own words involves not only your mind but also your body in the process of learning. The more physical senses you use in learning, the stronger the neural trace in your brain (p. 96).

From Pauk's discussion it is clear that the act of physically engaging with the material through the act of speaking and the motivation to retain the information are the crucial elements in moving the information from your short-term memory to your long-term memory. So if I wanted to remember that the most common cause of hypothyroidism is Hashimoto's disease, I would say aloud, "What is the most common cause of hypothyroidism? Hashimoto's disease is the most common cause of hypothyroidism." As you will see, recitation works, but there are no shortcuts: you have to want to learn the material and you have to explain it back to yourself.

Consolidating Your Notes

Many students find it helpful to consolidate the notes from their lectures and their reading into summary sheets or note cards in preparation for a test. The advantage of consolidating one's notes is that all of the information is in one place, which may make it easier to study. If you have chosen to consolidate your notes using note cards, go over your reading and lecture notes and extract each of the key concepts and terms that you need to know for your exam and place the concept or term on one side of the note card and an explanation on the backside of the card. If you have chosen to consolidate your notes using a summary sheet, divide your sheet in two with the concepts or terms on the left side and the explanation on the right side. An item on the front of your note card or on the left side of your summary sheet might look like this:

The kidneys' role in maintaining body pH

The right side of your note card would have the following information:

The kidneys regulate body pH by (1) decreasing NA+ ions, (2) holding onto hydrogen ions, and (3) secreting sodium bicarbonate.

You will need to go through all of your reading and lecture notes extracting the key concepts and terms that you will have to know. Most students find it easier to make note cards or summary sheets on a weekly basis rather than waiting for the period before the exam to create them.

Studying

Your goal in studying for your test in nursing school is to learn the material beyond the point where you know it: you want to master the material. You want to know the material as if someone's life depends on it and, indeed, someone's life probably will depend on it. Keep the importance of what you are doing in mind as you study. As discussed, you are not studying so that you can get an *A* or impress your professor. You are studying so that you are prepared to promote, maintain, and restore the health and well-being of the patients you will provide care for as a nurse. This is your motivation.

Real-World Snapshot 14-1

Advice for Students Who Are Struggling to Pass Tests

The first thing I tell students who are having trouble passing their exams in nursing school is: practice test questions and study the rationales. Many students who are having difficulty with test questions in nursing school are too focused on memorizing content. I advise them to worry less about memorizing and focus on understanding how to think critically and apply the information that is discussed in class and in their textbooks. One of the best ways to do this is to do test questions—at least five a day—from a NCLEX book (or if money is an issue, from their nursing textbook and the CD-ROM or Web site that accompanies your textbook [most do]) and then very carefully look at the rationale for the correct and incorrect answers to those questions to understand not only what the right answer is but why that answer is the right answer. Look at why the wrong answers are wrong, too. If you get them all wrong, do not get discouraged. Just keep working at it. Learning to think critically and apply the information that you learn in nursing school is a process, and you will get better with time and practice. I have found this successful in numerous students.

Jeanne Ruggiero, PhD, RN, APN-C
Assistant Professor, College of Nursing
Seton Hall University

Unless you have a photographic memory you are probably going to have to go through your note cards or summary sheets repeatedly to master the material. As with taking notes in class or reading assigned material in your textbook, you will approach the study of your note cards or summary sheets actively and systematically. You cannot just flip through the note cards or and hope that the material sticks—you have to get into it. If you condensed your test materials using note cards you will read the front side of the card aloud and try to answer the question in your own words. After listening to your answer, flip the card over and compare and contrast your answer with the answer on your card. Think about how the answers are different: Did you miss a detail? Are you using the terms correctly? How can you get yourself to remember the correct answer in the future? Would a mnemonic device help (see

Sidebar 14-4)? Would it help to draw a diagram? Read the correct answer to yourself aloud. Now put the correct answer in your own words. Repeat the process with the next card. If you are using summary sheets, cover the right side with a blank piece of paper.

As you go through your consolidated notes and start to learn the information, make a pile of note cards or highlight those items that are especially troublesome for you. Focus on your weaknesses, but remember your goal is to master the material so that, ultimately, you will have no weaknesses.

Other Study Tips

- Test yourself—Once you think you have mastered the material, find someone reliable to quiz you on your consolidated notes. If you have really mastered the material you will be able to retrieve the information on your consolidated notes without much trouble.

- Start studying early— Making the information that you will be exposed to in nursing school stick in your long-term memory requires time. As discussed, your preparation for tests begins on the first day of the semester. Plan on learning a little bit of material every day with time left for repetition.

Sidebar 14-4

Mnemonics

Mnemonic devices provide a structure or organizing framework for information that enhances memory. There are a number of different mnemonic devices that many students find useful. Two of the most commonly used are acronyms, or first letter mnemonics, and acrostics, which are a series of words, lines, or verses in which the first letters form a word or phrase.

For example, to remember the risk factors for osteoporosis, some use the acronym of *ACCESS*.

ACCESS:
Alcohol
Corticosteroid
Calcium low
Estrogen low
Smoking
Sedentary lifestyle

An acrostic mnemonic to remember the progression of a physical exam is "I'm A People Person":

Inspection
Auscultation
Percussion
Palpation

There are hundreds of these types of mnemonic devices, and many of them can be found on Web sites like www.medicalmnemonics.com

- Keep your study sessions short—Most students have difficulty studying for more than 15–20 minutes at a time, so plan on frequent study breaks. In addition, you will get more out of your studying if you schedule several 60–90 minutes study sessions rather than one marathon study session.
- Learn from the rationales—Many nursing students have trouble with nursing exams because they memorize facts and prepare for knowledge-based questions; however, most nursing exams are focused more on application questions. Studying practice test questions that come with the textbook (or on an accompanying Web site) and paying close attention to the rationales that accompany these questions will help improve your ability to handle application questions.

For some students studying in a small group or with a partner helps in mastering study material. Studying in this manner has two benefits. First, you are able to hear how someone else understands a concept and how it compares with your understanding. Second, explaining the material to a peer will enhance your understanding. While forming a study group has benefits, it is important that you initially study the material on your own. It is a waste of everybody's time—and can wreck your confidence—to find yourself in a study group in which you or your study partner does not know the material.

Group Study Tips

- Study on your own before studying in a group.
- Keep the group limited to no more than five people. For some students a study partner is better than a study group.
- Make a plan for how you are going to study, how long you are going to study (no more than 90-minute sessions), and what you are going to study before meeting.
- Set ground rules for study session (e.g., no cell phone conversation during study session).
- Make sure the study meets your needs. If you feel like the group's level of commitment to learning is not close to yours, do not continue to participate.
- If being in the group makes you feel anxious or frustrated, do not continue to participate.

Real-World Snapshot 14-2

Study Groups Are Not for Everyone

I have found that study groups are not always the best way for students to learn the material they need to learn in nursing school. In fact, for some students, study groups can be a distraction and can diminish learning. One factor that influences the value of a study group is how well the students in the study group have prepared individually for the material the group intends to study. In addition, there is some evidence multiple study sessions with peer-to-peer study groups do not improve learning. Consequently, in our program, we advise students interested in joining study groups to study independently before meeting with the study groups and then plan on meeting with the study group once before the exam. The study group should also be small enough so everyone has a chance to interact. A good size typically is three or four people.

Jane Kurz, PhD, RN
Associate Professor, Department of Nursing
Temple University

Real-World Snapshot 14-3

Starting a Study Group

Study groups are a very good way for students to save time and to work collaboratively at learning what they will need to know as a nurse. However, not all study groups are created equal, and students have to find the type of study group that is right for them. Start communicating and bonding with your classmates as early in your education as possible. Join your Student Nurses' Association, attend social gatherings sponsored by the school, and so on. Meet other students, and inquire about study groups or start one of your own.

Jeanne Ruggiero, PhD, RN, APN-C
Assistant Professor, College of Nursing
Seton Hall University

Multiple Choice Exams

Most of your tests in nursing school will be multiple-choice exams. Multiple-choice questions, like the kind you will see in nursing school and on the National Council Licensure Examination (NCLEX), consist of a *stem*, which is a partial statement, and several sentence endings (see Example 1), or a direct statement (see Example 2). One of the options is the correct answer and the other options are *distractors*. The ability to distinguish the distractors from the correct answer depends mostly on mastering the material; however, as with most other activities in nursing school and nursing, having a systematic approach improves efficiency. In this section, discussion is provided on improving your exam-taking techniques. The question stems were adapted from *Nursing 436: Clients with Complex Health Problems* (available at http://www-unix.oit.umass.edu/~helene/Nclexfinal.htm).

Example 1: Incomplete statement

A 54-year-old client with a history of kidney disease was started on Quinidine (a drug that decreases myocardial excitability) to prevent atrial fibrillation. The nurse is aware that this drug, when given to a client with kidney disease, may:

a. cause cardiac arrest.

b. cause hypotension.

c. produce mild bradycardia.

d. be very toxic even in small doses.

Example 2: Direct statement

The major complications of myasthenia gravis are myasthenic crisis and cholinergic crisis. As a nursing student caring for a patient in crisis, which of the following is most essential to your nursing care?

a. Weakness and paralysis of the muscles for swallowing and breathing occur in either crisis.

b. Cholinergic drugs should be administered to prevent further complications associated with the crisis.

c. The clinical condition of the client usually improves after several days of treatment.

d. Loss of body function creates high levels of anxiety and fear.

Read the Questions Before Looking at the Options

Always read the stem thoroughly and carefully before looking at the options. Determine what you believe the correct answer to be before looking at the options. However, even if you think that you know the answer, read all of the options carefully. As you read the options cross out those answers that you know to be incorrect. Remember that the correct option is the "best" or "priority" option; there may be other options that appear to be correct, but you are looking for the best option for *that* question. If you are unable to identify the correct option after several seconds of careful thought, move on to the next question. Your goal is to answer all of the questions that you are sure of first, and go back and struggle with the more difficult ones after you have gone through the test once.

Don't Fall for the Exotic or Unfamiliar

If one or more of the options associated with a question looks unfamiliar, this option is most likely a distractor. Take confidence in what you know. For example, look at the question below that might be on a pediatric theory exam in nursing school:

You have taken the history of a 15-year-old girl who has a Body Mass Index (BMI) of 19. The girl reported an inability to eat, induced vomiting, and severe constipation. Which of the following would you most likely suspect?

Sidebar 14-5

Taking Exams: All the Words Matter

In taking nursing exams, students really have to understand the English language and realize that all of the words in the question and the choices matter. Every word in the question is there for a reason, and some students make the mistake of reading past the question or reading past the choices and adding their own words and ideas. For example, a student may have a question relating to a patient with low hemoglobin and, realizing that women tend to have lower hemoglobin levels than men, look for choices that apply to women even though the gender of the patient was never indicated. I do not recommend that nursing students look for curveballs or trick questions. Read each test item carefully and focus on comprehending what question is being asked and not on what you think is being implied.

Carol Carofiglio, PhD, RN
Nursing Faculty
Helene Fuld School of Nursing In Camden County

a. Anorexia nervosa

b. Bulimia

c. Diverticulosis

d. Hypercalcemia

Maybe the correct answer does not jump right out at you, but at least two of the options (c & d) should seem out of place and should be eliminated. In your readings, class lectures, and preparation for this exam, it is highly unlikely that you would have reviewed any content referring to diverticulosis and hypercalcemia because they are not common in the pediatric population. In addition to staying focused on the subject matter of the course, stick with the basics. In designing their tests, most of your professors in nursing school are interested in assessing whether you understand the basic concepts of the course. Consequently, if you see obscure or unfamiliar options, they are most likely distractors. Keep in mind the advice given to new clinicians to guide them away from making an obscure diagnosis when a simple diagnosis is more likely, "When you hear hoofbeats, think horses not zebras." Use this advice to improve your test taking.

Focus on Negatives and Absolute Words

Negative words such as *not* or *except* affect the truth of an answer and call for your attention. Make sure that you circle or highlight these words, and consider carefully how they affect the validity of statements. In addition, absolute words such as *most, least, never, none, always, all, every, best,* and *worst* require special attention (circle or highlight) when they are in the stem or the options. These words imply that the statement must be true 100% of the time and may indicate a false answer. Look at the sample question below:

> While attempting to draw blood from a patient who is positive for AIDS, a colleague has just suffered a needlestick. Which of the following is the most important action for the individual to take?
>
> a. Get an HIV test immediately.
>
> b. Start prophylactic AZT treatment.
>
> c. Start prophylactic Pentamide treatment.
>
> d. Immediately start psychological counseling.

You should have circled *most* in the stem and *immediately* in the options A and D. Focusing on these words provides clues as to which of the options are distractors. Pauk (1984) emphasized that students should be very wary of absolute words in the options and went as far as to suggest that if one had to guess, then one should first eliminate all the options that contain absolute words. Regarding the sample test question above: for option A, you might not remember exactly how long it takes to convert to an HIV-positive status, but you probably know that it does not happen immediately, so you can take that option out of consideration. For option D, while you know that psychological counseling may be important, it is not more important than reducing the likelihood of acquiring HIV, so you can take that option out of consideration. This leaves options B and C and from your class lectures, reading, and test preparation, you can feel confident in choosing B as the correct answer.

Eliminate the Silly Option

Writing test questions is a time-consuming and challenging task, and sometimes it is difficult to come up with four good options. Consequently, out of desperation, frustration, or a combination of the two, many of your professors may include a silly option. For example, here is a question from an exam I gave in a research methods course:

Hypothesis testing occurs most frequently in which type of studies:

a. Qualitative studies

b. Quantitative studies

c. Both qualitative and quantitative studies

d. The Olympics

Even if you were unsure about whether hypothesis testing occurred in quantitative or qualitative studies (the answer is quantitative), you could be certain that it does not occur in the Olympics, and option D can be discarded from the options. In your NCLEX and other exams that have been standardized, you will not encounter silly options; if one of the options appears silly or foolish on a standardized exam, read it over again carefully.

"All of the Above" Is Correct More Often Than Not

As stated above, writing test questions is challenging, and many professors run out of steam, which can work to your advantage. An option with "all of the above" means that if you can find two of the options that are correct, you can choose all of the above. Look at the example below from an anatomy exam:

> The diencephalon is:
>
> a. located just above the brainstem.
>
> b. composed of the hypothalamus and thalamus.
>
> c. the location in the brain where sensory data first arrive.
>
> d. all of the above

You may not recall that the diencephalon is composed of the hypothalamus and the thalamus; however, you do remember that the diencephalon is located above the brainstem and is the location in the brain where sensory data first arrive. Consequently, you can confidently choose option D. However, just because all of the above is one of your options on a test, you must continue to approach your test taking systematically. It is still important that you read all of the options carefully and make sure that all of the options pertain to the question.

Pay Attention to Options That Look Similar

As you are taking a test, you want to ask yourself for each question, "What is being tested in this question?" Most test makers are trying to assess a specific content area with each test question, and the better you are able to determine what that area is, the better off you will be. For example, in look-alike options, as seen below, the test maker is usually tipping his or her hand as to what is being tested.

> The nurse administers indomethacin to a newborn with patent ductus arteriosus (PDA) to:
>
> a. open the ductus arteriosus.
>
> b. close the ductus arteriosus.
>
> c. prevent infection.
>
> d. increase heart rate.

When two options are included in a test that are similar with the exception of a word or two, you can often eliminate the other option(s) (after reading them carefully) and focus your attention on the two options that are look-alikes. In the question above the focus of the question is to assess whether you know that indomethacin is used to close the ductus arteriosus (option B). However, if you were totally unsure as to the role of indomethacin in PDA and you had to take a guess, you would probably want to eliminate options C and D and focus on options A and B.

General Test-Taking Tips

- Do not run out of time—Many students have made the mistake of underestimating the number of questions on an exam and rushing at the end to finish. To avoid making this type of mistake go through the exam and determine how many questions are on the exam. In addition, determine whether there are types of questions other than multiple-choice questions such as short answer or essay—on the exam that may be worth more points. It is in your best interest to be strategic in how you take the exam, so you will want to allocate a greater proportion of time to these questions.
- Don't rush—While you want to be sure that you do not run out of time, you do not get any extra points for being the first person to submit the exam, so don't panic if one of your peers turns in his or her exam well ahead of you. In fact, if you have an hour to take the exam, plan on taking the full hour.
- Don't be afraid to change your first answer—Chances are that you have been advised to "stick with your first answer" when taking multiple-choice exams. A substantial amount of research has been conducted on this topic over the past 70 years, and most studies show that the majority of answer changes are from incorrect to correct, and most people who change their answers usually improve their test scores (Kruger, Wirtz, & Miller, 2005). Consequently, if you have doubts about an answer that you have chosen, go ahead and change it.
- Review your exam before submitting—You will not be able to evaluate which questions you have doubts about if you do not allocate some time to review the exam before submitting it. Make sure you leave a few minutes to go back over the exam. In addition to reviewing the questions you are not sure about, make sure that you have not left any questions unanswered and there are no stray marks if using a scantron system. Make sure you wear a wristwatch; there may not be a clock in the room or it may be wrong.

There are some great resources on test preparation and test taking on the Internet. Included below are some Internet sites with additional information on test taking:

- TesttakingTips.com—www.testtakingtips. com/test/index.htm
- Study Skills Self-Help Information—http:// www.ucc.vt.edu/stdysk/stdyhlp.html
- Bucks County Community College—www. bucks.edu/~specpop/tests.htm

References

Kruger, J., Wirtz, D., & Miller, D. T. (2005). Counterfactual thinking and the first instinct fallacy. *Journal of Personality & Social Psychology, 88*, 725–735.

Nursing 436. Comprehensive nursing 1: Clients with complex health problems. (2007). Retrieved November 14, 2007, from http://www-unix.oit.umass.edu/~helene/Nclexfinal. htm

Pauk, W. (1984). *How to study in college.* Boston: Houghton Mifflin.

APPENDIX A

Additional Recommendations and Anecdotes

This appendix includes the additional recommendations, guidance, and anecdotes that I gathered from my nursing colleagues that do not specifically address getting the most out of nursing school. Although this content did not fit cleanly into one of the previous chapters, it will be valuable (or at least humorous) to prospective nursing students, nursing students, and those students who are on the brink of leaving nursing school and are ready to enter the profession of nursing.

Getting the Most Out of Clinical

For many students, the clinical practicum is one of the biggest challenges of nursing school, so it is not surprising that the faculty members that I interviewed for this book had a substantial amount to say about getting the most of the clinical practicums. Because all of these recommendations and anecdotes are valuable and have the potential to help nursing students, I have included them below.

Develop Cultural Competence

Cultural competence begins by thinking about how you perceive yourself and how that influences what you see when you look at another person. It also involves overcoming those preconceptions and getting in touch with how individuals respond to your behavior. While it is important to understand and be aware of what the predominant health beliefs or dietary practices may be in a certain culture—for example, it is helpful to know that because a Hindu person may be vegetarian, you do not want to be offering them prime rib—you have to connect with each individual *as an individual*. No matter their background, you have to figure out who that person is by asking questions, listening, and understanding their experiences. It comes down to respecting differences, and you can't do that without listening to them and learning about them, and that happens one on one.[1]

Create Miniature Care Plans

Here is one way for students to gain practice in applying the nursing process and thinking critically in a clinical setting. In most nursing programs students receive their clinical assignment at least 12 hours before their clinical day. Once you receive this assignment and you know who your patient is and some of the problems involved with that patient, I recommend taking some time to develop miniature care plans. In these miniature care plans you will assume (because you haven't met the assigned patient yet) a nursing diagnosis (e.g., ineffective airway clearance related to chronic obstructive pulmonary disease [COPD]) and generate as many nursing interventions as you can think of for that patient. Make sure to include all that you feel needs assessing. As I emphasize with my students, it is important that you develop these miniature care plans before the clinical day, when you are free from the stress and noise of the clinical floor and it is easier to think clearly. During the clinical day, when you have a little down time or are not sure if you are utilizing your time effectively enough, you can refer to this miniature care plan and make sure that you are implementing and evaluating the nursing interventions that you planned (in the privacy and quiet of your home) to do.[2]

---

1. Nanette Sulik, MSN, RN
Clinical Instructor, Department of Nursing
Rutgers, The State University of New Jersey

2. Laurie Karmel, MSN, RN
Clinical Instructor, College of Nursing
Rutgers, The State University of New Jersey

Get Comfortable

Much of my time is spent guiding students in becoming familiar with and comfortable receiving a verbal report from the nurse caring for their patient. I suggest becoming familiar with information contained in each system (neurologic, cardiovascular, respiratory, gastrointestinal, genitourinary, and pain) in order to identify and clarify missing information. This functions to help the student interact with the nurse and to gain more information serving as the baseline in patient assessment.[3]

Take Initiative

It is not uncommon for students to be in clinical groups in which there are 8 or more students, and it is hard for the clinical instructor to divide his or her time equally. Frequently, the students who receive the most attention from the clinical instructor are those who are having the most difficulty (the squeaky wheel gets the grease). While clinical instructors have to get students who are having difficulty "up to speed," most clinical instructors are willing and eager to make extra efforts on behalf of motivated students. However, students have to show initiative and identify themselves to the clinical instructor as a motivated and goal-oriented student through their words (e.g., telling the clinical instructor what they are interested in) and actions (e.g., showing up early and being prepared).[4]

Overcome Embarrassment

Students are nervous about doing health assessments on patients, especially those of the opposite gender, prior to starting clinical. To ease this anxiety I remind students that they are not assessing a patient (including the genitalia) because they *can* (that is where the embarrassment comes from), they are assessing a patient's genitalia because they *have a clinical reason and clinical responsibility that relates to the nursing process*. I remind students that as nurses we are guided by the nursing process and the assessment serves as a baseline of information. Students need to understand that every assessment they make and every interaction they have with patients can contribute to the nursing process and the nurse's role in promoting, maintaining, and restoring the health of patients.[5]

3., 4., 5. Laurie Karmel, MSN, RN
Clinical Instructor, College of Nursing
Rutgers, The State University of New Jersey

Take the One Hundred Dollar Approach
(Cost Management Awareness)

In the beginning of each clinical rotation I point out to students that on every hospital floor there are examples of supplies being wasted. I pretend to have an imaginary $100 that is being "tapped" every time someone on the floor does something wasteful. For example, when a nurse hangs an intravenous (IV) solution or tubing without labeling it, the expiration date is unknown and hospital policies require that it be discarded and replaced. To remind students of the importance of using supplies efficiently, I make reference to my imaginary $100 every time we identify inefficient use of resources on the floor by saying, "That's coming out of my $100." However, I also use my one hundred dollar approach to remind students that clinical is about making mistakes and learning from those mistakes and, while sometimes costly, clinical learning experiences are worth it. For example, when the sterile field is compromised because a student dropped his hands below his waist or turned his back on the sterile field, it is embarrassing for the student and costly because a new sterile field has to be set up; however, as I tell students, these types of experiences are "worth my 100 dollars" if the student has learned something and will be unlikely to make that mistake again. It also serves to demonstrate hospital employees' responsibilities and involvement in cost efficiency.[6]

Avoid Getting Too Wrapped up in Technical Skills

During their clinical rotations many nursing students become obsessed with practicing technical skills such as performing tracheotomy care, putting in Foley catheters, and changing wound dressings. Students need to remember that the focus of clinical is not to master the performance of technical skills—there will be plenty of time for that once you are employed as a nurse—your focus should be on learning to apply the phases of the nursing process (assessment, diagnosis, planning, implementation, and evaluation) while incorporating the skills in caring for patients and developing the cognitive and interpersonal skills you will need as a nurse.[7]

6., 7. Laurie Karmel, MSN, RN
Clinical Instructor, College of Nursing
Rutgers, The State University of New Jersey

Be Prepared for Pediatric Rotations

It is easier to make mistakes in administering medications to children than adults for a variety of reasons, such as the medications have to be diluted, and children vary so much in weight. This means that giving medications in the pediatric setting can be especially nerve-wracking for students, clinical instructors, and the parents of the pediatric patients who are often on the pediatric unit. Consequently, in pediatric rotations you *must* be sure of what you are doing. This means that you might want to spend some time in the clinical learning lab at your school to review the skills and knowledge you will need in the care of pediatric patients before you begin this clinical rotation.[8]

Look for Learning Opportunities in the Clinical Setting

Nursing students need to take a small picture view and a big picture view when they are in clinical practice settings. What do I mean by a small picture view and a big picture view? The small picture is that you have to provide care to the patients who have been assigned to you. However, in the big picture, nursing students should also be aware of the other problems that patients in that clinical setting are experiencing. For example, the patient currently assigned to you may have congestive heart failure while your peers may have patients with other health problems. Go back and read about those problems because you may be assigned to one of those patients and, while you may have to do more reading about patients with those kinds of problems, at least you will be a step ahead. Even if you are not assigned one of those patients, this knowledge will improve your practice as a nurse.[9]

Express Gratitude and Appreciation to Nurse Preceptor

Most nurses working on most patient care units in hospitals where nursing students receive the majority of their clinical experiences already feel overburdened by the

---

8. Joy Atkins, MA, RN
Adjunct Instructor, Department of Nursing
Rutgers, The State University of New Jersey

9. Randolph Rasch, PhD, RN
Professor and Director of the Family Nurse Practitioner Specialty
Vanderbilt University School of Nursing

number of tasks they have to complete on units that are crowded with patients and their families, nurses, and other hospital personnel (e.g., physicians, respiratory therapists, and social workers). While nursing students do not mean to be burdensome, they increase the workload for nurses who take on students by serving as preceptors. In my experiences as a clinical instructor I found that some of the nurses seemed like they felt forced into taking students and, in these instances, the student did not benefit much from the arrangement because the nurses did not slow down for the student or spend much time helping the student make sense of what was happening with a patient. Nursing students can improve relationships with nursing preceptors and diminish the likelihood that nurse preceptors will feel unacknowledged by showing these individuals, who are not compensated for precepting students, how much they appreciate their efforts. I am not suggesting that students buy their preceptors gifts, but verbally expressing thanks to the preceptor, demonstrating an eagerness and readiness to learn, and helping the preceptor out whenever possible are likely to improve nursing student–nursing staff relations.[10]

Be Conscientious about Clinical Expectations

I teach community health clinicals. Just like in the other clinicals, community health instructors expect students to (1) have basic nursing knowledge (e.g., to know how long an opened bottle of insulin can be kept refrigerated before it expires), and (2) to be able to perform the basic nursing skills they learn prior to beginning their community clinical experiences (e.g., how to administer a subcutaneous injection). Unfortunately, due to the sequencing of clinicals, sometimes students "get rusty" and forget the basics by the time they get to community health, which is often taken toward the end of the nursing education. Students have to take responsibility for retaining the basic knowledge and skills as they acquire new knowledge and skills. Most nursing schools have nursing skills and physical assessment labs where students can go to learn and review the basic (and more complex) nursing procedures that they may

10. Cynthia Ayres, PhD, RN
Assistant Professor, College of Nursing
Rutgers, The State University of New Jersey

have to perform in their community health rotation. Additionally, students have their nursing textbooks that they should review.[11]

Do Not Do Anything That You Are Not Sure Of

Students need to remember that safety comes first. I tell students that if there is some procedure or medication that they are not sure of they should wait for the clinical instructor. Do not feel pressured to take any actions you are not certain of.[12]

Overcome the Fear Factor

If possible, students should try to get hands-on experience working with patients before starting clinicals. There is a huge difference in the clinical starting point for students who have gained clinical experience by taking care of patients working or volunteering in a hospital setting and those who have not. Students who have clinical experience in providing hands-on care to patients with devices like Foley catheters, IV tubes, and monitors have gotten over the "fear factor" of putting their hands on patients and working around these devices. In turn, these students are more comfortable than their counterparts in performing such tasks as collecting vital signs and giving a quick bed bath. When students are comfortable doing the basics of patient care, such as bed baths, the clinical instructor can teach them how to assess skin integrity during the bed bath and relate that to nutrition, fluid intake, and laboratory findings and the possibility of dehydration or overhydration. The clinical instructor can also show the student how these findings relate to the clinical picture. For these students the focus is not on getting over the anxiety of providing a bed bath but on the assessment that can take place during the bed bath.[13]

Remember—You Know More Than You Think

Too many nursing students think, "I am only a nursing student. I don't know anything." In fact, nursing students know way more than they think they do. Here is

---

11., 12. Henry Soehnlein, MSN, RN
Clinical Instructor, College of Nursing
Rutgers, The State University of New Jersey

13. Laurie Karmel, MSN, RN
Clinical Instructor, College of Nursing
Rutgers, The State University of New Jersey

how I know this to be true. On the first day of clinical I usually ask my students to talk about the fears and anxieties they have as they prepare to begin clinical. Typical responses include: "I do not know what I am doing," "I do not know what I am going to do," and some students even admit "I am scared of you." On the last day of clinical I ask the students to think about the fears and anxieties they had on that first day, and I ask them to discuss what they learned. Invariably, students realize in retrospect that they had already learned all the information they needed going into clinical and that what they learned in clinical was how to pull it all together. For example, I do not teach students about electrolytes and what that means to the body. I do not teach students about the circulation of the heart and what happens when that circulation is altered. They learned it in anatomy and physiology and their other classroom coursework. What they do not know as nursing students is how to gather the subjective and objective information to facilitate making an evidence-based, clinical decision that benefits the patient. That is what my role is as the clinical instructor: I teach students how to apply the nursing process.[14]

Remember—Your Clinical Time Is Precious

In nursing school you have a limited amount of time on the clinical floors and, consequently, while you want to be helpful to the staff on the unit, you should not be performing trivial jobs or "scut work" (e.g., retrieving medicine from the pharmacy, taking specimens to the lab). If you find that you are being asked to perform these kinds of tasks, discuss this with your clinical instructor. Your judgment in prioritizing hands-on interactions will be respected.[15]

Remember—You Can Handle the Hard Stuff

Being an obstetrical (OB) nurse for 20 plus years has brought me much joy and personal and professional satisfaction. There is nothing more rewarding than helping to bring a new life into the world. I have also seen sadness though, when a family loses a baby and grief ensues. And while I encourage my students to consider OB nursing as a career choice, I do emphasize that we do not always have happy outcomes.

14., 15. Laurie Karmel, MSN, RN
Clinical Instructor, College of Nursing
Rutgers, The State University of New Jersey

Most of the students are excited after seeing a birth and say they would like to become OB nurses. Of course there are those students who have programmed themselves to believe they would only like to work in the emergency department (ED) or operating room and those who don't care for babies.

Then there are those students who are fearful and say "Wow, I didn't realize you are caring for *two* patients when you are taking care of a patient in labor!" Others are more insightful and say "Wow, you are really taking care of a whole family when you are taking care of a woman in labor!" Then there are those who comment "How do you do it? How do you take care of a Mom when she loses a baby? I could never do it!" Many of the students comment that they would never become an OB nurse solely for that reason. I tell the students that it is not uncommon for people to avoid these patients on the floor, including sadly, the nurses.

One semester the students and I were on the postpartum unit. I did not assign them to care for a patient who had a fetal demise because it was early in the semester, and they were not ready to care for patients who have experienced a perinatal loss—or so I thought.

As the evening progressed and the students were completing their assignments, I saw one of the students come out of the room of the patient who had experienced the perinatal loss.

The student and the staff nurse were deep in conversation, went to pick up items in the supply room, and went back into the patient's room. At the end of the evening, after reviewing my students' documentation, I sent them off to the solarium to wait for postconference. That student came out of the patient's room with the nurse, and I heard the nurse thank the student.

As we walked to the solarium together, the student said to me "I know I said I would never take care of a woman who lost a baby, but she needed me."

As we engaged in postconference and the students shared their experiences, I thought "What made the student feel that this patient needed her?" That student gave report last, telling us about the patient, the patient's history, and the fact that she noticed many of the nurses were avoiding that patient. She heard the nurses say they felt "uncomfortable," especially since most of them had healthy children of their own. After she finished the care for her assigned patient, she asked the nurse if she could go in with her to see this patient. As a tear rolled down her cheek, she explained to us "I went in and held her hand and spoke with her. She just wanted someone to listen to her and let her cry. I know because I lost a baby myself. Everyone was afraid and didn't know what to say to me or know what to do for me.

One nurse, though, sat with me for a very long time and held my hand while I cried. She encouraged me to hold my baby. I'm forever grateful that she was on duty that night. She made such difference for me. In turn, I hope I have helped this patient as well."

That certainly gave the students something to think about! Pulling the student aside after postconference, I told her that she will make a wonderful nurse. I know—I was one of those patients who experienced a perinatal loss.

My advice to nursing students is to be open minded and learn as much as you can in each area of nursing. Do not program yourself into believing that the only place for you is in one specialty—you never know where you may be needed.[16]

Get the Facts

One of the problems I have found is when students arrive in the acute care setting, especially the medical–surgical floor, the nursing staff are focused on making sure that nonpriority tasks such as bed baths are completed. A student's first order of business upon arriving on the floor is to verify what they received in report and to do a health assessment including a set of vital signs. For example, if a student receives report from the nursing staff that the patient assigned to him is receiving 5 liters of oxygen by nasal cannula and the patient is, in fact, receiving 10 liters of oxygen by nasal cannula, this needs to be reported to the clinical instructor. If a patient is supposed to be NPO (nothing by mouth), then there should not be a food tray in the room.[17]

Men in Nursing

I know many men who would be excellent nurses and love the profession of nursing; however, the thought of nursing school is a psychological hurdle. One of the

---

16. Patricia Coyne, MSN, RN
Instructor-Maternity Nursing
Cochran School of Nursing
Dedicated to the memory of my daughter, Lauren Nicole.

17. Jeanne Ruggiero, PhD, RN, APN-C
Assistant Professor, College of Nursing
Seton Hall University

reasons that I wrote this book was to help these men get over the psychological hurdle of nursing school. Many of these men may not know men (or women) who have gone through nursing school or they may be uncomfortable in asking about nursing school. I have tried to provide these men with an insider's view of nursing school and demystify the institution so that they understand what happens in nursing school and get over the psychological hurdle. The faculty members that I interviewed in developing this book share my belief that increasing the number of men in nursing is good for the healthcare system and good for nursing. The recommendations they have provided will help men get the most out of nursing school so that they can make meaningful contributions to the healthcare system and the profession of nursing.

Men in Nursing—Interacting with Patients

This is a generalization, but male students tend to interact differently with patients than their female counterparts. I think this is because, in our society, females are socialized to be more "warm and fuzzy, touchy-feely," and that is how we connect to those who we do not know. Men, on the other hand, have to find other ways to connect with others, and many have developed a great sense of humor that they can use clinically. It is a gift, and I have seen many male students use humor to put patients at ease.[18]

Men in Nursing—Stop to Ask for Directions

Some nursing students, more often men, I have taught are reluctant to admit that they do not know something (in the same way that many men will not pull over and ask for directions when they get lost). They want to prove that they are competent and feel that it is a weakness to ask a question or two. This impedes learning. These types of students take pride in feeling that they can figure something out clinically, but it is important to remember that you are dealing with a real person, and as the instructor I need you to know what you are doing or we need to talk.[19]

18., 19. Nanette Sulik, MSN, RN
Clinical Instructor, Department of Nursing
Rutgers, The State University of New Jersey

Men in Nursing—Cultural Barriers

Another issue that nursing students who are men should be aware of is that some-times female patients of various cultural backgrounds (e.g., women who are Muslim) have beliefs that make it impossible for them to have men provide personal nursing care practices such as bathing. Nursing students who are men should not take this per-sonally. Likewise, male patients of various cultural backgrounds cannot have fe-males care for their personal needs. I cannot overemphasize the importance of learning the practices of different cultures. And if you don't know, please don't be afraid to ask. Most individuals will appreciate your respect and willingness to pro-vide them the comfort of adhering to their cultural practices.[20]

Men in Nursing—Don't Get Railroaded

I have worked with so many great nurses who are men. One piece of advice I have for men who are considering what they will do in nursing after completing their ed-ucation is: do not get railroaded into working in the emergency room or a critical care setting if that is not what you want to do. Male nurses should not feel pressured to work in the emergency department where their strength is valued in dealing with patients who are violent or under the influence of drugs or alcohol. Men should feel free to pursue their own interests in nursing.[21]

Men in Nursing—You Are Not the Designated Lifters

Nursing students who are men need to know that they are not the "designated lifters" on the unit. On too many occasions I have seen the nursing staff make unreasonable requests of male students like, "Can you take this patient down to the morgue?" Male nurse students need to be aware, while it is important to be helpful to the nurs-ing staff, they are there to learn just like their female counterparts and that their clin-ical time should not be spent moving around heavy patients.[22]

---

20. Nanette Sulik, MSN, RN
Clinical Instructor, Department of Nursing
Rutgers, The State University of New Jersey

21., 22. Jeanne Ruggiero, PhD, RN, APN-C
Assistant Professor, College of Nursing
Seton Hall University

Assuming the Professional Role

Although the focus of this book has been on getting the most out of nursing school, a few of the contributors had some recommendations and anecdotes that will help students as they prepare to make the transition from nursing school student to nursing professional.

You Will Not Know Everything

Many students are under the impression that after they graduate from nursing school they will know everything they need to know to practice as a nurse: this is a misguided view, and students with this view need to recalibrate their goals. Your goal is to know how to practice. This includes: (1) knowing how to interact with patients and make accurate assessments; (2) knowing how to teach and provide information that your patients need; (3) knowing how to find the information you need to make evidence based clinical decisions; (4) and knowing when to refer your patient for further consultation.[23]

Control Is an Illusion

Part of our professional role as nurses is to understand what we can control and what we cannot possibly control in the lives of our patients. In most situations, we have very little control over what our patients know, do, and think, and we have to understand the limitations of our role or run the risk of driving ourselves crazy. Our role as nurses is to figure out where our patients are heading and to prioritize what we do in terms of that particular patient. For example, we cannot teach a patient who has just found out that he or she has Type I diabetes everything about the disease. For some of these patients you can teach them to administer their own injections, and for some you can get them all the way up to thinking about the diet; however, in all cases you have to think about the resources the patient has to work with in terms of social support, motivation, cognitive skills, and so on, and decide how to continually adapt your teaching based on how the patient responds.[24]

23., 24. Randolph Rasch, PhD, RN
Professor and Director of the Family Nurse Practitioner Specialty
Vanderbilt University School of Nursing

Begin Your Practice by Watching

As a nursing student and a new nurse, take every opportunity to observe and listen and evaluate the social dynamics of the unit you are on. Think about the actions that your colleagues have taken, and think about what you would have done differently if you were in their situation.[25]

Find Time to Laugh

Nurses, like other healthcare professionals who work with patients and families experiencing illness, have to deal with pain, loss, and sadness as part of their job. This can be stressful, which is why it is so important (and this begins in nursing school) to make time to share the happy and good experiences that you experience as a nurse. When funny things happens on the unit—like the error in communication that results in a 65-year-old patient giving you a semen specimen rather than a urine specimen— share this with your colleagues. Everyone needs a laugh, and providing opportunities for each other to laugh during the shift is one way we take care of each other as nurses.[26]

Master Entry-Level Knowledge

When you are taking nursing exams, and when you get around to taking your National Council Licensure Examination, remember that what professors and boards of nursing want to determine is: do you know what you need to know as an entry-level nurse? Consequently, when you are taking nursing exams, eliminate those alternatives that do not reflect the kinds of knowledge that entry-level nurses would possess.[27]

Anticipate the Odd Days

New nurses are expected to absorb and synthesize an incredible amount of information. Sometimes this makes it difficult to process what may seem like simple instructions. For example, I remember instructing a newly graduated nurse named

---

25., 26., 27. Elizabeth Ann Atkins, MA, RN
Clinical Director
Kennedy Health System

Karen who worked on the medical–surgical floor I managed that a stool specimen had to be collected from one of her patients. Because the physician who wrote the order wanted the stool specimen only every other day, I told Karen that she should only collect the stool specimens on "odd days." Karen agreed, and I didn't give our conversation another thought until 3 days later when I reviewed the patient's chart and noticed that there was no record of a stool specimen being obtained from Karen's patient Mr. Smith. Later that day I said to Karen, "I just noticed that you have not gotten Mr. Smith's stool specimens yet." She replied, "You know I was thinking about it and today is just not an odd day. Everything is just running as smooth as I could hope for. I will see how things go tomorrow, but I am hoping that things go as well as they have today and I do not have to collect it then either."[28]

Interview with a New Nurse

When I interviewed new nurses for employment I would always give them clinical scenarios to see what kind of clinical decision-making skills they had. In my interview of one nurse I said, "You go to see your patient, and all of sudden he grabs his chest and quickly becomes unconscious. What are you going to do?" The nurse pauses for a moment and then replies slowly and sincerely, "I am going to be awfully scared."[29]

Share Your Knowledge

Nursing is empowering. Your knowledge base is vast. There are others within the healthcare team that could benefit from your interpretation of your patient's status. There are others learning as you are. Share your knowledge. It is empowering and rewarding.[30]

28., 29. Elizabeth Ann Atkins, MA, RN
Clinical Director
Kennedy Health System

30. *Laurie Karmel,* MSN, RN
Clinical Instructor, College of Nursing
Rutgers, The State University of New Jersey

INDEX

Boxes, figures, and tables are denoted by b, f, or t following the page number.

A

AACN (American Association of Colleges of Nursing), 23

Abbreviations, 99*b*, 100*b*

Academic background for admission, 40–41

Academic dishonesty. *See* Dishonesty

Accreditation, 30–31

Accu-Chek, 201–202

Acute care settings, clinical time in, 190–193

Adapting to change, 186

Administration of nursing programs, 36, 37*f*

Admission to nursing school, 39–58
 academic background for, 40–41
 application process, 42–48, 50
 denial of, 48–50
 interview for, 45–46
 letters of recommendations for, 46–48
 parents of young children or infants, timing of, 41

personal statement/essay for, 42–45, 53–58

person-based qualities for, 41–42

Adults, course on nursing care of, 60

Advice for students having difficulty, 68, 222

Aged, course on nursing care of, 60

Aiken, L. H., 25

Air Force Academy and cheating scandals, 183

"All of the above" as exam answer, 229–230

American Association of Colleges of Nursing (AACN), 23

American Nursing Association on benefits of baccalaureate degree, 26

American Psychological Association (APA) format, 161–162, 164, 166

Anatomy and physiology course, 63

Anxiety *See* Stress

APA format and guidelines, 161–162, 164, 166